What in the World

Is Going On?

What in the Gut Is Going On?

Five Key Elements to Master Your Hormones

Dr. June E. Stevens

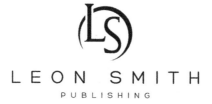

LEON SMITH
PUBLISHING

ISBN: 978-1-957972-85-5

I dedicate this book to my sister Jeannie.
You are my hero and my best friend. Your display of unrelenting strength,
courage, and perseverance while dealing with debilitating Crohn's disease
has inspired me to become the very best doctor I can be and to share all that
I have learned with others.

Table of Contents

Part One
What You Need to Know

CHAPTER 1

CHAPTER 2

CHAPTER 3

CHAPTER 4

CHAPTER 5

Part Two
What You Need to Do

CHAPTER 6

CHAPTER 7

Acknowledgments

Writing a book is hard. In fact, it was much harder than I imagined it would be. Speaking always seems to come naturally to me, whether it is one on one with patients in my office, leading a group in a classroom setting, or lecturing to large audiences in a convention center, and I assumed writing a book would as well. I was wrong. I think better on my feet than sitting on my butt at a computer. Writing this book challenged me in more ways than I imagined, and I am truly grateful for the lessons learned during this process.

However, completing this book would not have been possible without the help and support of some important people in my life:

My editors and Babypie Publishing. I absolutely could not have done this without you. I am a speaker, not a speller. I extend my greatest thanks to you and all your work to make this book come to life.

My teachers and mentors, Dr. Decker Weiss, Dr. Timothy Schwaiger, Dr. Paul Anderson, Dr. Thomas Kruzel, and the late Dr. Walter Crinnion being chief among them, for establishing the foundation on which I was able to build. Thank you for sharing your passion, wisdom, knowledge, and skills. Without you, my career would not be where it is today, and this book would not have been possible.

My many colleagues and friends who were there to talk, respond to emails, share ideas, provide feedback, act as a sounding board and, most of all, offer support and encouragement in times of frustration during this past year of COVID-19 isolation. I am so thankful to you all.

My countless patients, past and present—thank you for challenging me each and every day to stay on top of my game. Working with you has taught me so much and inspired me to share what I have learned with as many people as I possibly can; hence, the birth of this book. Thank you for helping me on my mission to move the world toward wellness.

My office manager, Annamarie, thank you for running such a tight ship at our office, affording me the most valuable of all necessary assets: time. Without it, this book would still be just one of my thoughts and not a true reality.

Finally, and most importantly, to my wife Melanie. I thank you for all the love, encouragement, and support you have provided me, not just while writing this book, but always. Thank you for being you. I am blessed and truly grateful to have you in my life.

A Note From Dr. June

When I first entered medical practice as a naturopathic doctor in 2005, I had no idea I would end up where I am today, writing a book on digestive health for hormonal balance. I had been a cardiac critical care nurse for fifteen years prior to attending medical school. At that time, I felt determined to become a naturopath cardiologist with my emphasis in women's cardiology. What I didn't realize was that the Universe had an even grander plan for me.

I absolutely love practicing naturopathic medicine. I feel so blessed to have discovered my passion and to live and work with it every day. I have been honored and privileged to work with thousands of patients within my practice over the years and look forward to continuing to do so. However, I began feeling as though I ought to be doing something more. I was having this increasing sense—call it *intuition* or a *gut feeling*—of something brewing inside of me. Something was eager to manifest, but I was not sure exactly what it was until I had my *aha moment.*

On May 14, 2018, I had my epiphany while listening to a speaker at a women's entrepreneur meeting. We all were encouraged to consider what lay outside the boundaries we often locked ourselves into based on our profession. What if we allowed ourselves the wider perspective of what she referred to as our *chosen vocation?*

Immediately, I knew what my gut had been telling me for the past few years: *You are an educator, June, and it's time for you to take that outside your office and outside the classroom. You need to step out and share your naturopathic wisdom and expertise with the world. No longer confine yourself to your practice. It's your time to branch out to promote greater health, which is so desperately needed in the world today.*

The vision of a book immediately came to mind. In that moment, all seemed crystal clear. I'm a doctor, but I needed to give myself permission to answer my second calling: fulfilling my role as a health educator on a grand scale. Immediately, I felt uplifted and free. I felt alive again. And then a bit of fear, self-doubt, and anxiety began to creep in. I already had a full medical practice. I asked myself: *How am I going to do this?*

My answer: *Trust yourself. Do not surrender to fear and self-doubt. Trust the Universe and surround yourself with those individuals who want to help you make this happen.*

The Universe intervened, all right. It placed the COVID-19 pandemic front and center. One of the positive sides of being in lockdown with events and activities cancelled for nearly a year was that I found something valuable: time to write my book. It's been quite a journey, and I'm grateful for the lessons I learned along the way.

My book is now in your hands. My hope is that the words I present in this book provide you with the information and knowledge—and thus, the power—you need to maximize your digestive health to balance your hormones and achieve your highest level of health.

Foreword

What in the Gut Is Going On? will improve your life! Its author, Dr. June Stevens, does such outstanding work in holistic medicine that we included her in a set of interviews with prominent experts in various domains. Those experts include a Pulitzer Prize-winning New York Times journalist, an Academy Award-winning Hollywood videographer, a leading nuclear engineer, an Olympic gold medalist figure skater, and more. The work these experts do is very important; however, Dr. June's highly innovative, ethical work might represent the most important expertise of all because she is at the forefront of a movement to reform medical care for the better.

Dr. June Stevens is a brilliant, holistic medical expert. She is an excellent example of "transformational giftedness," which means she uses her impressive knowledge and talents to make the world a better place. This book will break readers free from the narrow-minded, shortsighted, superficial, rigid thinking that can limit perceptions of healthcare. Those who read it will move to the front of the paradigm shift that will enable them to address the causes of their health problems instead of just the symptoms.

Don Ambrose, PhD
Creative intelligence researcher
Editor of The Roeper Review

Introduction

There is a silent epidemic of hormonal imbalance—let's refer to it as *ED*, better known as *estrogen dominance*—and it's affecting the quality of life for millions of women today. Conventional medicine has little to offer these women except medication. Antidepressants, antianxiety medications, sleeping pills, or birth control pills—all are used in attempts to ease their symptoms.

Treating symptoms is not the answer. Addressing the underlying cause is the solution. The missing link to maintaining hormone balance for so many women today is impaired gut function. Yes, that is correct. Gut health—which includes the optimal function of your gallbladder, liver, and microbiome—is a major driving factor for your overall health, yet few are aware of the impact the gut has on our hormone balance. Restoring gut function through diet, lifestyle, and detoxification is your first step on the quest to restore and maintain hormone balance.

For the past thirty years, there have been hundreds of peer-reviewed research articles published in medical journals supporting the idea that lifestyle plays a significant role in the risk for disease.

Research shows these factors significantly impact your health:

- Food
- Sleep
- Stress management
- Exercise
- Thoughts you focus on

The question: why is this information not more apparent and accessible to the people who so desperately need it and want it?

The answer: because there is no *magic pill* and therefore no money to be made by the medical industry with lifestyle medicine.[11]

I am pleased to say a paradigm shift is happening. Lifestyle medicine is taking hold and the health and wellness industry is quickly establishing a solid foundation. You, the healthcare consumer, are a driving force in the process of moving medicine from a *sickness* to a *wellness* model.

As a naturopathic doctor, I am pleased and honored to play a part in such a major transformation in healthcare. Join me as I share with you the science-based research portraying the significant role gut health plays in maintaining hormone balance and your overall health. The research is there. It is just not getting out to the general public fast enough.

My mission is to share this information with you, to educate and empower you to be your own advocate and maximize your gut health, restore your hormonal balance, and improve your overall health. I want to inspire you to share this information with others so we can move the world toward wellness together.

Part One

What You Need to Know

Chapter 1

A Silent Epidemic

There is a silent epidemic affecting the quality of life for millions of women worldwide today, and no one is talking about it. Women are experiencing a hormonal imbalance that I refer to as *ED*, short for *estrogen dominance*.

You may be more familiar with ED standing for erectile dysfunction—but that is not what I'm talking about here. I am talking about estrogen dominance and how it is affecting women at an unprecedented rate. Some sources, such as the *New York Post* and hormone health expert Christine Mullin (MD, FACOG, IVF Director at Northwell Health Fertility), say 50–80 percent of women will be negatively affected by hormonal imbalance, and sadly, a majority will suffer in silence.[2,3] Women often come to their healthcare provider with complaints of *just not feeling well* and comment *something doesn't feel right* in their body.

The challenging symptoms of hormonal imbalance are variable (see Table #1), often overlap, and, in most cases, tend to manifest slowly and progressively. Unless your healthcare provider takes time to truly listen to you and put the pieces of your health picture together, hormonal imbalance is often overlooked, mistreated, or untreated. When conventional medicine does turn to treatment, it unfortunately has little to offer women aside from prescribing medications as attempts to alleviate their presenting symptoms.

Many women are prescribed antidepressants or anti-anxiety medications to address their emotional fluctuations, sleeping pills for their disturbed sleep, and even low-dose birth control pills to reduce their symptoms. To make matters worse, some women are told their symptoms are a part of the *normal aging process* and are left untreated.

Think about these questions:

- Why are healthcare practitioners simply treating symptoms and not identifying and addressing the underlying cause?

- Why are these symptoms so prevalent in women today?

- What can be done to help women get back their quality of life?

I have written this book to address and answer these questions.

Symptoms are your body's attempt to get your attention and let you know when something is out of balance. Symptoms are not meant to be suppressed; they deserve to be addressed. Conventional medicine treatments are ineffective for hormones, have unwanted side effects, and, in some situations, may worsen the presenting symptoms.

Why? Because the underlying cause is not being addressed and the whole person is not being treated.

Restoring and maintaining hormonal balance is a complex process because your hormones do not work independently. Instead, they work synergistically. Let's take a closer look at the interrelationship between our estrogen, progesterone, thyroid, and adrenal hormones.

I see an increasing number of women of varying ages in my clinic, not just perimenopausal, presenting with symptoms of estrogen dominance, and they feel miserable. Their estrogen-dominant state is negatively impacting their mood, sleep, energy, and weight. Many had sought treatment for their symptoms elsewhere prior to coming to my office and were disappointed and or frustrated with their treatment options and outcomes.

Estrogen dominance is a significant health issue, and if left untreated, it can contribute to many of the chronic diseases that are prevalent today:

- Hypothyroidism
- Gallbladder disease
- Weight gain
- Insulin resistance and diabetes
- Hypertension
- High cholesterol
- Blood clots
- Strokes
- Cardiovascular disease
- Cancer

Due to the frequency of estrogen dominance I see in clinical practice, I decided this information must be shared on a much larger scale. I believe women deserve to know what's going on with their bodies. I find women are eager to understand what's happening within their bodies, and most of all, they want to know what they can do to bring their hormones back into balance and get their lives back on course.

The chart below is a tool I use with my patients in clinical practice to help simplify the complexity of hormones. Take a moment to review the chart below. Which symptoms are you experiencing?

Table #1: Hormone Symptom Evaluation Tool

	High Estrogen	Low Estrogen	Fluctuating Estrogen	High Progesterone	Low Progesterone	Fluctuating Progesterone	High Testosterone	Low Testosterone	High Cortisol	Low Cortisol	Fluctuating Cortisol	High Thyroid	Low Thyroid	Fluctuating Thyroid	High DHEA	Low DHEA
Acne					•		•								•	
Anxiety	•		•		•				•		•					
Arthritis (joint pain)					•			•								
Bladder symptoms		•						•								
Brain fog		•			•					•			•			
Breakthrough bleeding		•			•											
Breast tenderness	•				•											
Cramping					•											
Diminished sex drive (libido)		•			•			•		•			•			
Depressed mood		•			•			•		•			•			•
Drowsiness				•												
Dry skin/hair		•											•			
Endometriosis	•				•											
Fatigue		•		•				•		•			•			•
Fibrocystic breast	•				•											
Fibroids	•				•											
Fluid retention/ bloating	•				•								•			
Food cravings					•					•						
Hair loss		•					•	•					•	•	•	

	1	2	3	4	5	6	7	8	9	10	11	12	13	14
Harder to reach orgasm		•			•			•						
Headaches	•		•		•	•		•					•	
Heart palpations		•										•		
Heavy/irregular periods	•				•									
Hot flashes		•	•		•			•						
Irritability	•					•	•		•					
Memory loss		•						•					•	
Mood swings	•				•									
Night sweats		•									•			
Nipple tenderness				•										
Sleep disturbances/insomnia		•			•		•				•	•	•	
Vaginal dryness		•						•						
Weight gain	•				•			•					•	

Each bullet point indicates a symptom that may be induced by the corresponding hormone levels.

What Exactly Are Hormones?

Your hormones are vital to your overall health and well-being. Although different hormones are examined and talked about independently, they work in conjunction with each other to regulate your metabolism. Metabolism is responsible for maintaining our body temperature, weight, and energy level. Hormones also support our body in growth and repair processes and play a critical role in modulating fertility.

Hormones are our body's signaling molecules and deliver information to our cells. Each of our hormones has a unique function within our body. They are produced and stored in the endocrine organs. When signaled by the brain, the endocrine organ releases its hormone locally and into the bloodstream. Once in the bloodstream, the hormone is picked up by carrier proteins and shuttled to their target tissue. When it arrives at the target tissue, the hormone binds to its receptor and tells the tissue what to do, when to do it, and for how long.

A symphony is a good analogy for hormonal balance. Hormones act in response to a signal from the brain. Symphony performers play music in response to cues from their conductor. Hormones act independently, and yet have a significant impact on one another. The same is true for symphony performers. Even though each plays their individual piece of music, together they play a part in a much larger performance.

Much like the symphony, precision and timing are critical with hormones. When they are balanced and working in harmony all goes well, but if one musician is off key or if the hormones are out of balance, the harmony is lost. For many women, the thought of trying to comprehend and navigate the complexity of hormones can be confusing and overwhelming, but women can feel when their hormones are out of balance—they simply do not feel well, and their quality of life suffers.

Women are desperately searching for answers and solutions to improve their quality of life. Finding answers and solutions within conventional medicine can prove challenging. Women are often left feeling frustrated as they continue to struggle through their health journey. However, there is hope. Stepping outside of the conventional medical model and into the alternative, or integrative, healthcare arena has proven to provide the answers many women have been searching for.

Naturopathic doctors, along with many providers trained in integrative or functional medicine, are far less likely to simply treat symptoms. Instead, we strive to determine the underlying cause of your unique situation. Your symptoms serve as a guide for us. We listen to your story to uncover the underlying common threads and work with you to identify the obstacles to you achieving better health. We assess for hormonal imbalances by using surveys, questionnaires, and functional laboratory testing. (We test saliva for adrenal and sex hormones levels and urine for sex hormone metabolites.)

We strive to help our patients achieve *optimal ranges* in their laboratory tests, as the so-called *normal ranges* have proven to be unreliable for many people. The majority of hormonal imbalances seen today are consequences of our lifestyle and surrounding environment, so we feel it's important to educate our patients on what they can do to restore and maintain their hormone balance. For many, hormones are out of balance because life is out of balance. Our goal is to provide our patients with tools and resources that empower them to become more proactive in their own self-care.

When I was in medical school at Southwest College of Naturopathic Medicine & Health Sciences, I learned about the six guiding principles of naturopathic medicine:

1. **Do no harm** *(primum non nocere)*: Naturopathic doctors choose the least invasive and least toxic treatment options necessary for each patient.

2. **The healing power of nature** *(vis medicatrix naturae)*: Naturopathic doctors recognize, respect, and support the body's inherent ability to heal itself.

3. **Identify and treat the causes** *(tolle causam)*: Naturopathic doctors seek to identify and a remove the underlying causes of disease rather than suppress symptoms.

4. **Doctor as teacher** *(docere)*: Naturopathic doctors strive to instill their patients with hope and knowledge and empower their patients to reclaim agency for their own health.

5. **Treat the whole person** *(tolle totum)*: Naturopathic doctors treat the whole person, not the disease, by addressing the physical, mental, emotional, spiritual, genetic, environmental, and social factors impacting a person's life.

6. **Prevention** *(praevenic)*: Naturopathic doctors promote overall health, wellness, and disease prevention.

The fourth principle of naturopathic medicine, *Doctor as Teacher*, is something I take seriously. I, along with my fellow naturopathic and functional medicine providers, support the belief that prevention is the best medicine and that educating our patients on self-care is the first step toward prevention.

Why Is Hormonal Imbalance Such an Issue?

Hormonal imbalance rarely occurs as the result of one cause. Most often it is due to a combination of factors that might include:

- Dietary habits
- Nutritional status
- Sleep cycles
- Stress levels
- Activity levels
- Lifestyle behaviors
- Medications
- Environmental toxicants

The good news here is that each of these factors is modifiable in ways that can promote, restore, and enhance hormone balance. The problem is that the necessary modifications are not being made. Not to focus on the negative, but we should pay more attention to statistics.

Research shows hormonal imbalances are on the rise. Cases of breast cancer in young women (under age forty) are increasing.[4] *Polycystic ovarian syndrome* (PCOS), the most common reproductive endocrine disorder in the United States, is also on the rise. Currently, it affects one in ten women in the United States and one in fifteen women worldwide.[5] Twenty million Americans suffer from thyroid disease, the majority being women. Obesity, along with all the chronic diseases now associated with it, is also on the rise worldwide.[6] Taking it one step further, the World Health Organization (WHO) declared in 2018 that chronic diseases (heart disease, diabetes, cancer, autoimmune diseases, and Alzheimer's) have now surpassed infectious diseases as the number-one cause of death globally.[7]

What is even more striking is that the chronic diseases seen today are caused by a very short list of lifestyle behaviors.

Topping this list are:

- Poor nutrition
- Lack of physical activity
- Tobacco use
- Excessive alcohol intake[8]

Here in the United States, some 80 percent of healthcare costs are related to chronic diseases, and 80 percent of these chronic diseases are related to lifestyle choices.[9] This brings us back to the importance of education and empowerment in order to support prevention and self-care.

For the past thirty years, hundreds of peer-reviewed research articles have been published in medical journals that support this fact: our lifestyle plays a significant role in our risk for disease.

Research shows there are multiple lifestyle factors that significantly impact your health:

- The types of food you eat
- The amount of sleep you get

- The stress you are under
- How much you exercise
- The environment in which you live

Why is this information not getting out to the people who so desperately need and want it? Because there is no *magic pill* that can fix it. Without the ability to manufacture a drug, there is no real money to be made by the medical industry.

The truth is crystal clear: Our lifestyle matters. The way we live our life and the daily choices we make—what we choose to eat, drink, think, and do—can lead us down a path toward illness and disease or a path toward health and wellness. Lifestyle medicine is the solution to the problem of chronic disease. Let's take the path to wellness together.

Identifying and treating the underlying cause of any illness or disease is needed in order to achieve a successful outcome. In order to effectively treat and, more importantly, prevent hormone imbalance from occurring in the first place, we need to determine the underlying causes. Unfortunately, when it comes to hormonal imbalance there are many contributing factors.

Some occurrences of hormone imbalance are induced by the use of medications, both over the counter (OTC) and prescription, or by an underlying medical condition. However, hormonal imbalances are most often induced by a combination of factors occurring over time:

- Dietary habits: what, when, how, and how much we are eating
- Lifestyle behaviors: activity level, alcohol, and tobacco use
- Stress levels: mood, mindset, and sleep cycles
- Toxic environments: jobs, hobbies, personal care products, cleaning supplies, and pollutants
- Impaired digestive health: malabsorption, dysbiosis, inflammation, and impaired elimination

Yes, that is correct: impaired gut function has now been linked to hormone imbalance.

I would venture to say that impaired gut function, induced by all the factors mentioned above, goes far beyond hormone imbalance and is the common thread within a majority of the chronic diseases seen today. Could it be that the solution to hormone balance rests in our gut?

The answer is yes.

Does Estrogen Deserve Our Attention?

Estrogen is most often thought of as a reproductive hormone because it is involved in maturation, fertility, and reproduction. And yet it does so much more. You have receptors for estrogen everywhere in your body. Estrogen plays a vital role in your metabolism and energy production. It supports and protects your cardiovascular health, bone health, and brain health and is often referred to as *the hormone of memory and cognitive function* for women. It is also responsible for regulating our cell growth and replication.

Now, the female body produces three types of estrogens: *estrone* (E1), *estradiol* (E2), and *estriol* (E3). During our reproductive years, our ovaries are the primary producers of both our estradiol and estrone, whereas our liver is the producer of estriol. After menopause, our adrenal glands take on the responsibility for estrogen production, along with our fat cells and gut microbiome.

A few words of wisdom for you ladies: consistently nourishing your adrenal glands is important because they are your natural backup system for hormone production after menopause. Healthy adrenals help support healthy hormones.

E2 is the estrogen that receives the most attention, as it is the predominant and most potent estrogen produced during our reproductive years, and it is the form most commonly prescribed for hormone replacement therapy. E2 is thought to be about ten times more potent than E1 and 100 times more potent than E3.[10] The challenges with estrogen arise when it is not balanced well with progesterone, or when it is inefficiently cleared out of the body. In either case, a state of *estrogen dominance* ensues.

Estrogen dominance contributes to conditions like weight gain, *premenstrual syndrome* (PMS), fibrocystic breasts, uterine fibroids, *endometriosis*, and cancers of estrogen-sensitive tissues (breast, uterus, or ovary). On the other hand, E1 is the predominant circulating estrogen in our body throughout our post-menopausal years. Because our ovaries no longer produce hormones in our post-menopausal years, E1 is produced mainly in our adrenal glands and fat cells. E1 can be interconverted to E2 by our liver and has the ability to stimulate estrogen receptors, but it is still weaker than E2.

Finally, there is E3—the least potent of all estrogens. E3 is typically found in very low levels in your body. The only time this is an exception is during pregnancy because the placenta produces high amounts of E3 throughout the pregnancy.

Despite the fact that the estrogens have varying potencies, they interact and influence each other within our body. This is why balance is key. Unfortunately, living in today's world can easily disrupt our estrogen balance, resulting in estrogen dominance. We are being exposed to higher levels of *exogenous*, or external, estrogens than ever before.

These exogenous sources enter our bodies through environmental exposures. *Xenoestrogens*, industrial and chemical compounds that are completely foreign to our body, are found in plastics, fragrances, and pesticides, which are all around us. Our inorganic food choices, animal or plant products, are contaminated with hormones or herbicides and pesticides. These are known to be hormone disruptors. To add insult to injury, many of us are unknowingly auto-toxifying ourselves through our own impaired gut function.

Yes. That is correct—your gut health and microbiome play a significant role in regulating estrogen, xenoestrogen, metabolism, and elimination. When impaired, our gut microbiome tends to recycle hormones, xenoestrogens, and toxicants rather than excrete them out of our body through our bowel. The recycled estrogens, xenoestrogens, and other toxicants then act additively with our own *endogenously*, or internally, produced estrogens, which contribute to a state of chronic estrogen dominance. And, as we now know, higher levels of estrogen can increase the risk for cellular growth, predisposing us to cancers.

What Is Estrogen Dominance?

Let's take a look at estrogen imbalance, but estrogen dominance specifically. The term *estrogen dominance* was originally coined in 1996 by Dr. John R. Lee in his book titled, *What Your Doctor May Not Tell You About Menopause: The Breakthrough Book on Natural Progesterone* (Warner Books, 1996). Estrogen dominance is a state within our body when our estrogen level is high in relation to our level of progesterone.[11]

This is a naturally occurring process in a woman's body as she transitions from perimenopause to menopause (see Image #1). The first hormone to naturally decline during this period is progesterone. By nature, a women's body is designed to have a balance of estrogen, which stimulates cell growth, relative to progesterone, which regulates cell growth. With the onset of perimenopause (as early as thirty-five years for some women) and progressing into menopause (typically between fifty and fifty-two years), this balance is disrupted as natural progesterone production begins to progressively decline at a faster rate than estrogen. This results in a relative excess of unopposed estrogen, or estrogen dominance.

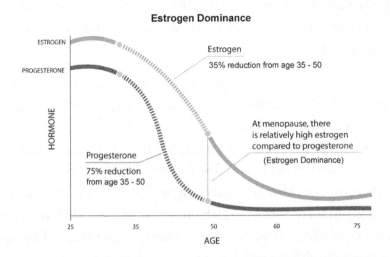

Image #1 – Estrogen Dominance

Due to our changing world and environmental exposures, women (as well as men and children) of all ages are at greater risk for developing estrogen dominance today than ever before. Why? We are all continually being exposed to external sources of estrogen, xenoestrogens, and toxicants resulting in the bioaccumulation of these sources within our bodies. Over time, this accumulation contributes to overall hormone disruption, including estrogen dominance.

In addition to environmental exposures, chronic stress also takes its toll on your hormone health, particularly in menstruating women. Living a fast-paced, high-stress lifestyle alters levels of your stress hormone, *cortisol*, which negatively affects your overall digestive function and leads to inflammation. Elevated gut inflammation can then inhibit the natural release of progesterone during a woman's menstrual cycle and directly contribute to the onset of estrogen dominance. I am seeing more and more such cases in clinical practice.

Every day, I work with women of various ages presenting with obvious symptoms of estrogen dominance.

They experience symptoms such as:

- Fatigue
- Weight gain—particularly in the hips, thighs, and abdomen
- Disturbed sleep
- Mood disturbances—such as irritability
- Foggy thinking
- Memory decline
- Headaches
- Digestive impairment
- Irregular menstrual cycles or worsening PMS—for those still cycling
- Fibrocystic breasts
- Fibroids
- Endometriosis
- Low libido
- Cancer—breast, uterine, ovarian

When I discuss with them the term *estrogen dominance*, most have never heard of it and have no idea what it means.

Patient education is always a large part of their treatment plan. Helping women understand their bodies and empowering them to become active participants in their own health is necessary to prevent the long-term consequences associated with estrogen dominance.

Estrogen Dominance and Your Thyroid

Many women suffer needlessly because estrogen dominance is often overlooked, unacknowledged, and unaddressed by conventional medicine. This poses significant health risks for women. Aside from unpleasant symptoms, estrogen dominance has far-reaching effects in your body, ranging from thyroid and gallbladder dysfunction to obesity and cancers.

Over time, it will only go from bad to worse. Excess or unopposed estrogen may induce a hypothyroid state. How does this happen? Well, estrogen stimulates our liver to increase its production of a protein known as *thyroid-binding globulin* (TBG).

If you recall, when a hormone is released into the bloodstream, the majority is picked up and bound to its specific carrier protein to be delivered to target tissues. In the case of thyroid hormone, more than 99 percent is bound by TBG, leaving only a small amount of active hormone available.[12] This is important because the free thyroid hormone, not the bound hormone, is the active hormone.

The problem arises when excess estrogen triggers the overproduction of TBG. Higher levels of TBG bind up too much of your thyroid hormone, rendering it inactive and unable to do its job. The end result is an induced hypothyroid state, which lowers our metabolic rate and leads to increased symptoms of fatigue, weight gain, and constipation.

To add fuel to the fire, this induced hypothyroidism further perpetuates estrogen dominance. How so?

1. While in a hypothyroid state, your liver receives less stimulation from the thyroid hormone, thus becoming less efficient at metabolizing estrogen and other toxicants, which furthers their accumulation and worsens estrogen dominance.

2. Hypothyroidism results in an overall reduction in bile flow, and inhibits the relaxation of the *sphincter of Oddi*, decreasing bile flow out the ducts and into the small intestine.[13]

3. Less thyroid stimulation to our gastrointestinal tract results in slower gut motility, contributing to constipation. Since one of the primary elimination routes for estrogen is through your bowel movements, any level of constipation contributes to more estrogen recycling and a worsening of estrogen dominance.

Have you ever wondered why hypothyroidism is so much more prevalent in women compared to men? Estrogen dominance may be a contributing factor.

Estrogen Dominance and Your Gallbladder

Over time, estrogen dominance contributes to gallbladder dysfunction as well. An excess of estrogen diminishes the gallbladder's motility. This decrease in motility leads to ineffective contraction and insufficient bile release. In addition, excess estrogen enhances the formation of cholesterol gallstones, which also may lead to insufficient bile release.[14]

Have you ever wondered why so many women in their forties and fifties (I will admit I am seeing it in even younger women today) have gallbladder issues or have had their gallbladders removed compared to men? Stay tuned! In Chapter 2, I will address the important roles your bile and gallbladder play in maintaining your estrogen balance.

Estrogen Dominance and Cancer

Honestly, the topic of cancer is huge and deserves a book all to itself, of which, there are many great ones. I recommend *Cancer: The Journey from Diagnosis to Empowerment* (Lioncrest Publishing, 2020), by Paul Anderson, ND, and *The Metabolic Approach to Cancer* (Chelsea Green Publishing, 2017), by Nasha Winters, ND. The point I want to stress here is this: estrogen is essential for our overall health and vitality, yet it often gets a bad reputation.

When the topic of estrogen comes up, most people are quick to think of its negative side—it causes cancer. This is not necessarily true.

What we do know is that unopposed estrogen may trigger unregulated cell growth, particularly in the estrogen-rich tissues of the breast, ovary, uterus, and endometrium, resulting in the increased risk of cancer.[15] We also know our progesterone balances our estrogen by regulating its effect on cell proliferation. I would further argue *endogenous estrogen*, in and of itself, is not bad. The *potential bad* arises when estrogen is not balanced well with progesterone or when it is inefficiently cleared out of the body.

Whether there is too much estrogen or too little progesterone, the outcome is the same: estrogen dominance. I would further venture to say the *true bad* comes as a result of xenoestrogens, chemicals, and other toxicants negatively impacting hormone balance and our body's ability to clear out both natural estrogens as well as the xenoestrogens. Over time, this estrogen dominance state can have deleterious effects on our overall health, cancer being one possible outcome.

Estrogen Dominance and Men's Health

Okay, ladies, I realize this book is intended for you. However, I feel compelled to take a moment to address the fact that men and children are also being affected by estrogen dominance. Why?

The same reasons apply:

- Additives to our food supply
- Hormone use in animal agriculture
- Toxic pesticides, herbicides, and insecticides use on our crops
- The use of plastic in our daily lives
- Our sedentary lifestyle

All these factors drastically impact our body's digestive health and hormone regulation. The increased exposure to these *xenobiotics*—chemical compounds foreign to your body—have proven to negatively impact the health and well-being of both humans and animals.[16] Despite this, they are still in common use today.

Since the 1980s, we have seen a sharp increase in the number of young men suffering with lower testosterone levels, and research shows environmental exposures, such as Bisphenol A (BPA), found primarily in plastics and heavy metals, such as lead and mercury, are likely contributing factors.[17] In addition, as men age into their forties, their testosterone levels decline as more of their testosterone is being converted into estrogen by the enzyme *aromatase*.

Aromatase is predominately found in fat cells, particularly in belly fat. This poses a vicious cycle in men: the more belly fat a man has, the more aromatase acts in his fat cells, which increases the conversion rate of testosterone to estrogen, further perpetuating belly fat gain and an estrogen-dominant state.[18]

Compounding this issue, our sedentary lifestyle has been shown to perpetuate weight gain and plays a role in the process as well. Much like elevated estrogen in women, elevated estrogen in men leads to a host of unpleasant symptoms and a heightened disease risk. Symptoms of fatigue, loss of muscle mass, low libido, mood decline, and erectile dysfunction are commonly experienced with both lower testosterone and higher estrogen levels. Long-term effects of higher estrogen and lower testosterone levels may lead to insulin resistance, increased cardiovascular risk, and a predisposition to an increased risk for prostate cancer.[19]

How Do I Know Whether I Am Estrogen Dominant?

As mentioned at the beginning of this chapter, estrogen dominance is a silent epidemic affecting millions of women worldwide. Many of these women know and feel something is out of balance in their body, yet they struggle to find answers, solutions, and support during their quest to get their life back on course.

In the conventional medicine arena, the causes of estrogen dominance are often lumped into three broad categories:

1. The use of exogenous hormones—birth control pills and hormone replacement therapy

2. Genetic issues

3. Lifestyle

Ironically, the only treatments offered to symptomatic women in conventional medicine include exogenous hormones, BCPs for younger women, and estrogen replacement therapy for menopausal women.

Remember: a woman's body naturally produces estrogen, progesterone, and testosterone.

So, is prescribing estrogen-only replacement therapy to menopausal women a wise idea?

I say not. When it comes to *hormone replacement therapy* (or HRT), progesterone and testosterone are essentially ignored. Additionally, conventional medicine pays little attention to genetics, until after cancer manifests. Genetics then become a larger topic of discussion as a course of treatment is mapped out. Discussion about lifestyle and the role it plays in hormone imbalance and cancer is nearly nonexistent in conventional medicine. This is a sad truth.

Is it any wonder why so many women feel lost and alone on their path to finding hormone balance?

I am on a mission to change this. Naturopathic doctors approach the prevention and treatment of ED from the complete opposite end of the spectrum. We start with lifestyle approaches first, as they are the most impactful on maintaining and restoring hormonal balance.

Research continues to show how influential our environment and lifestyle choices are on our genetics and whether they are expressed, such as being turned on and resulting in disease. Our approach is to guide our patients as they take a serious look at their diet, lifestyle, stress, and environment.

In some cases, genetic testing is done to identify potential risk. Functional medicine testing is often done to evaluate the patient's digestive health, liver health, nutritional status, and hormone levels. Our goal is to identify the obstacles to your health and hormone balance in order to treat the cause. At times we may prescribe HRT, yet only after the foundation—your diet and lifestyle—has been addressed. Even then, we are more likely to prescribe compounded, bio-identical hormone replacement therapy in clinical practice if, and when, it's indicated.

To help you determine if you, too, may be experiencing estrogen dominance, take a few minutes and complete your self-assessment by evaluating these five items:

1. Symptom List: Revisit the provided chart above. Are you experiencing symptoms of low progesterone? Excess estrogen? How about low thyroid?

2. Diet Diary: Are you eating all organic foods, whole foods, and only wild caught and free-range animal products? Do you limit dairy and gluten?

3. Habits and Hobbies: What are your bowel habits, sleep habits, and exercise habits? What is your intake of alcohol, caffeine, sugar, and tobacco?

4. Environments and Exposures: How clean is the air you breathe, the water you drink, and the food you eat? How about your personal care products, household cleaning supplies, and use of plastics both at home and at work?

5. Existing conditions and medications: Do you have, or suspect you have, any liver, gallbladder, or digestive issues? Are

you regularly taking any prescription or over-the-counter medications?

Testing for Estrogen Dominance

The good news is that hormone testing is available. Hormone levels can be evaluated using a sample of venous blood, capillary blood, saliva, or urine. The challenge lies in deciding which testing method is best for you in your given situation.

For menstruating women, the day and time of sample collection is important to interpret results correctly and accurately. If you are taking hormone replacement therapy (oral, sublingual, topical, or vaginal), the method of collection (blood, saliva, or urine) is important for accurate results.

As with any laboratory testing, there are limitations along with pros and cons. In conventional medicine, venous blood sampling—blood taken directly from the vein—is considered the gold standard method of testing hormone levels. The pros? It is fairly quick and easy, and results are available in just a few days. The cons? It is invasive, requires going to a doctor's office or lab, and only provides a quick snapshot of where the hormone levels were at that specific day and time.

One limitation with blood testing is that it measures the levels of protein-bound hormones. These hormones are bound to the carrier proteins *albumin* or *sex hormone-binding globulin* (also known as SHBG). These are not free hormones, so the serum level may not be reflective of the amount of free hormone exerting its effects at the actual tissue level.[20]

Saliva testing is a more useful way of measuring levels of free hormone. The pros? It requires very little preparation and can be done from the convenience of your own home on a designated day and at a specific time. This is particularly useful if you are still menstruating. The cons?

The results are not recognized by conventional medicine, and it takes about two weeks to get the results. The limitation is that saliva testing does not allow for the evaluation of hormone metabolites.

In order to evaluate how well your body is metabolizing and excreting hormones, urinary testing of hormones is most useful.[21] The pros? It is done at home on designated dates and provides the levels of both hormones and their hormone metabolites. Why are metabolites important? The evaluation of hormone metabolites provides a lens to view how well your body is metabolizing hormones and determines how efficiently enzyme pathways are functioning.

This is important, as these enzyme pathways can be easily influenced by our nutritional status, diet and lifestyle choices, and environmental factors. In the end, the evaluation of hormone metabolites allows for a determination of potential risk. The cons? Urinary hormone testing tends to be more expensive and requires a bit more preparation. In some cases, a first morning sample is needed. In other cases, a twenty-four-hour collection may be necessary. Sometimes a urine dip—a dried urine sample—needs to be taken at designated times within twenty-four hours.

One major limitation to all forms of hormone testing is that xenoestrogens are not reflected in the test results. Xenoestrogens can significantly impact how our body utilizes, metabolizes, and excretes hormones. That said, hormone testing provides valuable information, but it does not replace the need for a detailed history and symptom evaluation along with a physical examination. For the best outcome, all these are considered.

How Do I Restore and Maintain My Estrogen Balance?

The solution to restoring and maintaining hormone balance in today's world may surprise you.

I hope it does.

The truth is this: The so-called *secret solution* has been, and continues to be, in plain sight. It has been right in front of our eyes, yet completely overlooked, up until now. The solution is the integrity of our gut health.

Yes, that is correct. It turns out gut health is one of the greatest predictors of your hormone balance, whether you are male or female, young or old. Research continues to support the fact that gut health is directly related to overall health, hormones included.

While you move into the next chapters, I will share with you just how important your gut health is to your hormone health, and what you can do to maximize your gut health and restore and maintain your hormone balance.

Who would have believed our lymphatic flow, bile flow, liver function, and intestinal flora or *microbiome* would determine our hormone balance?

Join me as I take you on a journey, chapter by chapter, so you, too, can discover what you can do to maximize your gut health, your hormones, and your life.

Chapter 2

_____

Your Lymphatics—The Forgotten Detoxification Organ

Patient Case Study: "Judy"

I first met Judy in December of 2018. She was a fifty-five-year-old menopausal woman attending post-graduate school and working full time as a physical therapist. She was having difficulty making it through her workday due to fatigue, very low endurance, joint aches, and a sensation of heaviness in her arms and legs. Her symptoms were severe enough that she was having difficulty getting up from a chair. Judy was suffering from impaired lymphatic flow.

During our initial visit I also learned she was experiencing a lot of digestive issues: frequent gas and bloating, indigestion, feeling full quickly, and constipation. On examination, I noticed the edema in her lower legs (thighs to feet) and the skin on her hands and forearms was very taut, making it difficult for her to bend her knees or clench her hand to make a fist.

She was not taking any medications, nor did she consume alcohol, tobacco, or excess caffeine. Although she was attempting to eat well (mostly organic foods) her diet was rich in dairy, eggs, and some gluten-containing products. We decided to get some lab tests done, as she had not had any testing done in over three years.

The good news was her thyroid and blood sugar levels were healthy. However, her inflammatory marker (hs-CRP) was elevated at 3.4 (a normal level is less than 1.0), her iron levels were low, and her urine organic acid test (OAT) revealed elevated levels of yeast, fungal, and bacterial metabolite markers. We started with treating her gut by eliminating microbes to reduce inflammation and get her bowels and lymphatics moving again.

Over the course of the next three months, Judy was a trooper. She adhered to a yeast-elimination diet and avoided all sugar, simple carbohydrates, fruits, and juices. Instead, she focused on non-starchy veggies, lean proteins, and healthy fats. She had a weekly lymphatic massage to support her lymph drainage and infrared sauna therapy to support her overall detoxification.

In addition to dietary modifications, she consistently followed a gut-restoration regimen consisting of bitters with meals to stimulate digestive flow, natural antifungal and antimicrobial herbs and a binding agent (activated charcoal) to eliminate the gut microbes and toxins, probiotics to replenish her gut flora, liver support to facilitate detoxification, and curcumin to aid in reducing inflammation.

At her three-month follow-up, Judy reported that the aches and heaviness in her arms and legs were gone. She actually performed squats in the office to show me how much better she felt. She was now having two or three bowel movements daily, her weight was down fifteen pounds, and her energy level was to a point where she was planning to work out with a trainer at the local YMCA.

According to Judy: "Getting my digestive tract and lymph moving has transformed my life."

What Is the Lymphatic System?

When thinking about the lymphatic system, most of us automatically think of lymph nodes and fighting infection. And yes—it's true lymph fights infection. The primary function of your lymphatic system is to transport lymph, which is a fluid containing white blood cells (T-cells,

B-cells, and *natural killer* or NK cells) to fight off infection in your body.

However, are you aware of the other key functions your lymphatic system carries out?

Your lymphatics support the absorption of fats from your intestinal tract. They play a critical role in regulating fluid balance in your body. They also aid in ridding your body of waste, toxins, and hormones. Yes, that is correct. Your lymphatics play a distinct role in detoxification. Think of your lymphatic system as a subsystem of both your circulatory and immune systems. When your lymphatic system is not functioning optimally, neither can your circulatory system. This leads to fluid accumulation and toxicity overload, which lead to inflammation and disease.

I liken it to this: Your lymphatics are responsible for doing a great deal of work behind the scenes. They serve as both a delivery system as well as the clean-up crew, so to speak. Yet our lymphatics get very little, if any, recognition for all the work they do.

You may be thinking: *Okay, so what does all this have to do with fluid balance and my hormone balance?*

Let's take a closer look.

Lymphatics and Fluid Balance

You've probably heard it said that our bodies are made up mostly of water. And this is true. On average, the adult human body is made up of 60 to 70 percent water.[22] The percentage varies depending upon the amount of lean body mass (muscle) compared to the fat mass a person has. Lean tissue retains more water than fat tissue; therefore the leaner you are, the higher body composition of water you are likely to have. Maintaining and supporting your body's fluid levels are essential to sustaining life. And the health of your lymphatics plays a unique and critical role in this balancing process.

As most of you are aware, the primary function of your vascular system is to deliver life-sustaining oxygen; nutrients, like electrolytes and amino acids; hormones; and blood cells to all your body tissues. At the same time, it removes metabolic waste products, toxins, hormones, and debris from your body tissues. This exchange process occurs in your body's tiniest blood vessels, known as *capillaries*. At the levels of the capillary, your nutrient-rich blood plasma diffuses through the arterial end of the capillary into the tissue, while the waste and debris from the tissue reabsorbs back into the capillary via the venous end. However, there is not an equal exchange of fluid during this process.

Not all of the fluid diffused out of the capillary is reabsorbed back into the venous end of the capillary. It is estimated that approximately twenty liters of plasma flow through your arterials every day, yet only seventeen liters are returned to circulation by way of your venous system. What happens to the remaining three liters of fluid (also known as *interstitial fluid*) left behind in the tissues? This is where your lymphatic system comes into play and regulates overall fluid balance and rids your body of waste.

Found in every region of the body except those not containing blood vessels (like the bone marrow and central nervous system, or CNS), the job of your lymphatic capillaries is to mop up these remaining three liters of interstitial fluid. This interstitial fluid contains not only fluid, but also cellular debris; pathogens, such as bacteria; plasma proteins; and hormones, which all need to be cleared from the body. Once the interstitial fluid is picked up by the lymphatic capillaries, now referred to as *lymph*, it begins its slow journey back into circulation.

Lymph is carried through a network of lymphatic vessels—filtered within the lymph nodes along the way, emptied into lymphatic ducts—and is eventually returned to circulation via your *right* and *left subclavian veins*. Without healthy, functioning lymphatics, the interstitial fluid would simply continue to accumulate around the cells within tissues, resulting in the buildup of cellular waste products and the development of tissue swelling—known as *edema*—and toxicity.

The Lymphatic System and Hormone Balance

You may be wondering: *What could the lymphatics possibly have to do with hormone balance?*

To have hormone balance, your body's natural detoxification processes must be functioning. Unfortunately, when the topic of hormones and detoxification comes up, everyone—including practitioners—skips over lymphatics and quickly jumps right to the liver. Sounds like a good idea, as the liver is thought to be our body's largest detoxification organ, but there is a big problem with this approach.

The lymphatic system needs to be open and draining well before a liver detoxification process is initiated. Otherwise, it's putting the cart ahead of the horse. It's not going to work well, and in many cases, it will backfire. What does backfiring look like? Simple: the body cannot tolerate the liver detoxification treatment and the patient's symptoms worsen or the patient develops new symptoms.

Think about it: The goal of detoxification is to move unwanted materials out of the cells to excrete them from the body. During this process, hormones and toxins are moved out of the cells and into the interstitial fluid. It is the job of your lymphatics to collect and return this fluid, along with the waste materials contained within it, back into circulation for eventual elimination from your body via your kidneys or bowel.

But if the lymphatic channels are blocked or congested and cannot flow to remove hormones or toxins, they end up being deposited elsewhere in the tissues, leading to redistribution of that waste. Therefore, assuring that the lymphatics—drainage pathways—and the *emunctories*—natural routes of elimination—are open and flowing is a critical first step in the detoxification process.

Considering the whole body, assessing for lymphatic congestion or stagnation before initiating detoxification is the only safe and effective approach. The key role your lymphatics play in this detoxification process is frequently forgotten, overlooked, and neglected. And, when ill functioning occurs due to lymphatic congestion or stagnation, hormone imbalance and toxicity manifest. Your lymphatics are a filtering and drainage system for your body. When the network of lymphatic vessels, tissues, and organs are all working together, your body is able to maintain fluid balance and remove toxins, waste, hormones, and debris to maintain overall homeostasis.

Lymphatic System at a Glance

Palatine tonsil
Submandibular node
Cervical node
Right internal jugular vein
Right lymphatic duct
Right subclavian vein
Thymus
Lymphatic vessel
Thoracic duct
Cisterna chyli
Intestinal nodes
Large intestine
Appendix

Left internal jugular vein
Thoracic duct
Left subclavian vein
Axillary nodes
Spleen
Small intestine
Aggregated lymphatic follicle (Peyer's patch)
Iliac node
Inguinal lymph nodes

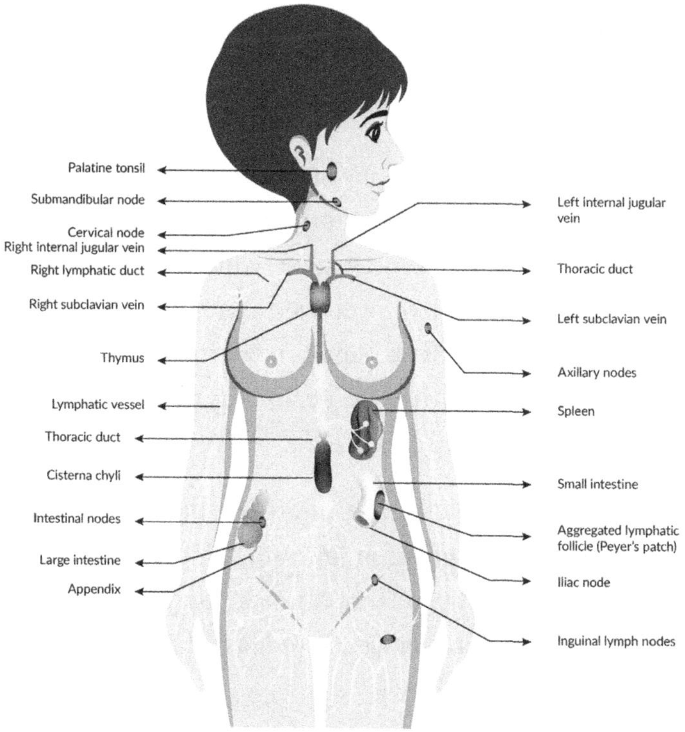

Image #2 – Lymphatic System at a Glance

What Is the Gut-Lymphatics Connection?

Aside from regulating fluid balance and removing waste, the lymphatics are also known for their role in immune function. This book is about the gut-hormone connection, so I'm not going to discuss the role that lymph tissue and organs play in immunity. However, one major component of your lymphatic system, known as the *gut-associated lymphoid tissue* (GALT), is worthy of discussion.

Why is GALT so important? GALT is found primarily in the small intestine and is the largest mass of lymphoid tissue found in your body.

This tissue provides massive amounts of lymphatic flow within your gut. Your GALT serves as your body's first line of defense against infection and invasion. Research clearly shows that our gut health is the gateway to our overall health, with more than 70 percent of our immune function stemming from our gut health.[23]

Any impaired digestive function can pose significant risk to your GALT, negatively impacting your hormone balance and overall health. Conditions, such as chronic constipation, which severely impedes your gut lymphatic flow; irritable bowel syndrome (IBS); small intestinal bacterial overgrowth (SIBO); small intestinal fungal overgrowth (SIFO); and food sensitivities, are becoming more common and are known to alter the integrity of your gut.

A breach in the integrity of the intestinal lining, known as *leaky gut syndrome*, or a dysregulation in your GALT can result in an inflammatory cascade. This inflammation is now understood to be the root cause of hormone imbalance, as well as all chronic diseases seen today.

What Makes Your Lymphatic System Unique?

Unlike your vascular system, which is driven by the pumping action of your heart, your lymphatic system relies solely on compression to continually propel your lymph and return it to your circulation. Even though your lymph vessels contain one-way valves to help prevent the backflow of fluid, they require ongoing compression in order to propel lymph in one direction, which is often upward and against gravity.

Where does this much needed compression come from? There are four primary sources:

1. Muscle contraction. This is why physical exercise and movement are so important.

2. Your respiratory pump. This is why deep breathing is so important.

3. Pulsations from nearby arteries. Lymph vessels tend to lie next to arteries throughout the body.

4. Peristaltic contractions of smooth muscle, both within the lymphatic vessels and the peristaltic actions within your gut. This is why constipation, SIBO, IBS, or any delayed motility can negatively impact lymph flow.

Unlike the pumping action of the heart, the lymphatic peristaltic activity can best be described as a very slow and gentle wavelike motion. The slow speed of peristaltic activity is important. If you recall, on average, there are approximately three liters of interstitial fluid recovered by your lymphatics every day. The slow wavelike motion allows time for lymph fluid to be filtered through your lymph nodes in order to remove pathogens before it is returned into circulation.

Referred to as *lymphatic congestion or stagnation*, lymph flow that is too slow will lead to fluid retention and toxicity. Please note I am not referring to lymphedema associated with the removal of or damage to your lymph nodes as a part of cancer treatment. What I am talking about is a sluggish lymphatic system induced primarily by lifestyle choices and behaviors.

How Do I Know Whether My Lymphatics Are Congested?

Unfortunately, there really are no conventional laboratory tests available that can reflect the status of lymphatic flow, nor are there any tests to determine how the lymphatic system impacts overall hormonal balance. The most accurate ways to determine if lymphatic congestion is present and how it may be impacting hormone balance are by evaluating your diet and lifestyle and listening to your body by tuning in to your symptoms.

The following are some of the most common signs and symptoms of lymphatic congestion I encounter in clinical practice:

- Feeling puffy, swollen, and stiff, especially in the morning
- Retaining fluid, or edema
- Gaining weight or having difficulty losing weight
- Feeling bloated
- Breast swelling with the menstrual cycle
- Menstrual cramping
- Brain fog
- Fatigue
- Dry and itchy skin or skin rashes
- Chronic congestion or infections: sinusitis, sore throats, colds, and ear pain or pressure
- Enlarged lymph nodes

What causes lymphatic congestion?

After reading the above list of signs and symptoms, you may find that you are experiencing many of them. If so, you are likely dealing with sluggish lymph flow. Now, there are many potential causes for sluggish lymph flow, yet in most cases it is brought on by a combination of factors, not just one. Below, I've listed some of the more common causes for sluggish lymph flow and suggestions for improving lymph flow.

Common causes for sluggish lymph flow:

- Lack of exercise or movement
- Dehydration
- Poor diet
- Lack of sleep
- Chronic stress
- Environmental toxins
- Constipation or gut inflammation

- Trauma or injury
- Infections
- Parasites

Common ways to enhance and improve lymph flow:

- Exercise
- Keep hydrated
- Modify your diet
- Sleep
- Reduce your stress level
- Limit restrictive clothing
- Dry skin brushing
- Lymphatic massage
- Hydrotherapy
- Sauna therapy
- Herbal medicines—*lymphagogues*
- Homeopathic drainage remedies

Historically, the Western medical community has neglected the lymphatic system and ignored the role lymph congestion plays in contributing to disease. Why? Let's go back for a moment and review the causes of lymphatic congestion and the ways to improve it.

Notice that most of the causes, with the exception of parasites and infections, revolve around lifestyle choices and behaviors. The best ways to restore or decongest lymphatics include lifestyle modifications and natural therapies.

That's correct: *Lifestyle medicine and natural therapies are not part of our Western medicine model.*

There are no pharmaceuticals to treat lymphatic congestion, so the condition *doesn't exist* in Western medicine. As a naturopathic doctor trained in Traditional Chinese Medicine (TCM), I am here to say that it does exist. In fact, it is more prevalent in today's society than ever before.

Our ever-increasing toxic exposures, combined with our high-stress and sedentary lifestyles, are directly contributing to lymphatic congestion. As you will read later (Chapter 7 provides you with twelve ways you can "liberate your lymphatics"), these same factors are also compromising gallbladder, liver, and microbiome function, inducing hormone imbalance and chronic disease. In clinical practice, educating patients on the importance of lymphatic health and incorporating lymphatic support measures as means to restore and maintain hormone balance are integral parts of the treatment plan. The severity of lymphatic congestion determines the level of intervention necessary to decongest your lymphatics.

As I prefer to say: liberate your lymphatics to harmonize your hormones.

Chapter 3

Your Gallbladder and Bile—
The Dynamic Duo

Patient Case Study: Alice

I first met Alice in April of 2017, when she came to my office concerned about her digestive health. She wondered if she had some food intolerances that had been affecting her mood and hormone balance. She shared with me that, in 2012, she had been hospitalized for a bout of severe abdominal pain, and her appendix and stone-filled gallbladder were removed.

Since her surgery, she had been self-treating with diet changes, probiotics, and digestive enzymes, yet noted ongoing gas and bloating with alternating constipation and diarrhea. Her symptoms intensified in 2016, after taking two rounds of antibiotics for a urinary tract infection. She was then diagnosed with colitis by her primary care doctor.

At the time of her initial appointment, Alice was still struggling with alternating bowel patterns, gas and bloating, yet had begun to experience episodes of anxiety and what she described as "a weird feeling lasting up to two days at a time," which seemed to be triggered by eating certain foods. She was eager to have a food sensitivity test done to see how she could change her diet.

I shared with her that it was not uncommon for women to develop digestive symptoms following gallbladder removal, as they tend to experience bile insufficiency leading to impaired absorption of fats, changes in bowel motility, and potential gut flora imbalances. I also shared with her that the two courses of antibiotics she had taken likely impaired her gut flora and gut function. Both can trigger changes in mood and brain function.

We moved forward with a food sensitivity panel. Because it takes about two weeks to get the results, we decided to go ahead and start a yeast elimination diet in the interim, as the likelihood of yeast overgrowth was high due to the use of antibiotics and removal of the gallbladder. I changed her digestive enzyme to one containing ox bile to support fat absorption, since she didn't have a gallbladder, and I changed her probiotic to one with a higher potency and containing Saccharomyces boulardii, which is helpful in the treatment of candida overgrowth.

At the time of her two-week follow-up, Alice had already experienced marked improvement: far less anxiety and less gas and bloating with the yeast elimination diet and supplement changes. Her results were, as we suspected, positive for candida. She was also found to be sensitive to gluten, dairy, eggs, and soy. The plan was to continue her candida elimination diet and eliminate her food sensitivities over the next eight weeks. We also included a few additional supplements: natural antifungals to eliminate the yeast, binders to remove toxins, and gut-healing nutrients to reduce inflammation and promote healing. I assured Alice we would address her concerns about hormones on her next visit, since the first step to restoring her hormone balance was healing her gut. Correcting her bile deficiency—which was important because hormones are eliminated through the bile—and restoring her gut flora—to prevent the recycling of hormones—were both necessary to support her hormone balance.

Why Are the Gallbladder and Bile So Important for Hormone Balance?

Much like our liver, which I will discuss in great detail in Chapter 4, our gallbladder is not considered to be a very *sexy* organ; therefore, no one really spends much time talking about it. Unfortunately, it is likely the most underappreciated organ in our body. In fact, in conventional medicine, the gallbladder is considered to be a *nonessential organ*, and we are led to believe we can live a completely healthy life without it. I disagree.

Yes, we are able to live without our gallbladder. But I would venture to say that we are not able to live as healthy a life without it.

The truth is, *cholecystectomy*, the surgical removal of the gallbladder, is one of the most commonly performed elective abdominal surgeries worldwide, with approximately 700,000 procedures occurring in the United States every year. Now, if that number did not get your attention, maybe this one will: of those people undergoing gallbladder removal, 40 percent, or 280,000 people, continued to experience long-term abdominal symptoms post gallbladder removal. This condition is so prevalent it has received its own name: *Postcholecystectomy Syndrome.*[24]

Think about this for just a moment: If the gallbladder is a nonessential organ, then why would we all be born with one in the first place? And why are there so many long-term complications associated with its removal?

Most of us think of the gallbladder as our body's storage container for bile. It is true the gallbladder provides a storage space for the bile produced within our liver, allowing it to concentrate and enhance its potency over time.

What happens when our gallbladder is not functioning properly due to conditions such as inflammation (*cholecystitis*), gallstones (*cholelithiasis*), common bile duct stones (*choledocholithiasis*), infections (*cholangitis*), or in cases where the gallbladder has been completely removed (*cholecystectomy*)? The answer is there is an inadequate output of concentrated bile. This is called *bile insufficiency*, and it is especially common in cases post gallbladder removal.

Bile insufficiency is an ever-increasing problem seen in clinical practice today. The challenge is that doctors of conventional medicine do not acknowledge this fact, nor are they appropriately addressing the long-term complications associated with it.

Over time, bile insufficiency leads to a host of digestive impairments and other major health challenges, including:

- Malabsorption of fats and key nutrients

- Altered intestinal pH balance

- Dysbiosis (intestinal microbial imbalance)

- Motility issues (contributing to constipation and diarrhea)

- Decreased ability to remove hormones, waste, and toxins from the body

Bile insufficiency directly impacts our hormone balance and contributes to estrogen dominance. I would take it one step further and say that it is directly contributing to the sharp increase in many of the chronic diseases we are experiencing. Not just here in the United States, but in our world today. One of my missions is to address this head-on by sharing this information widely. I intend to stress the importance of getting back to the core of gut health and the role it plays in maintaining our hormone health and the prevention of chronic disease. It starts with our bile. Yes, that's correct—our bile. Let's take a closer look.

Why Bile?

Let's start with what bile is. It's a yellowish, slippery fluid consisting mostly of water, bile salts, cholesterol, *phospholipids* (mostly *phosphatidylcholine*, or PC), and bile pigments (mostly *bilirubin*). Each of the bile constituents plays a role in keeping bile healthy. The bilirubin in our bile, a byproduct from the natural process of breaking down red blood cells, is what gives our urine a yellow color and our stool a brown color.

It's time I ask you an important question: Do you take the time to look at and evaluate your bowel movements?

You may be surprised to know that the color, texture, consistency, size, shape, frequency, and odor of your stool can tell you a great deal about the health of your gut. For the record, as an ND, I ask my patients many poignant questions about their bowel movements. But now, back to bile.

Another constituent of bile is PC, which is a major component of all our cell membranes. The function of PC within bile is to keep it thin and slippery by keeping the cholesterol more soluble, which ultimately decreases the risk of gallbladder sludge and gallstone formation.[25] In addition, PC protects the cells lining the bile ducts and intestine from the harsh scrubbing actions of our bile salts.

I want to take a moment and clarify what can sometimes be a confusing topic: Bile, bile acids, and bile salts are different terms often used interchangeably. But they are not actually the same thing. Bile acids fall into two categories, either primary or secondary.

Primary bile acids are synthesized from cholesterol by our liver cells (*hepatocytes*). When combined or conjugated with two amino acids, called *taurine* and *glycine*, they become bile salts. Bile salts are the components within our bile that act as detergents to emulsify the fats we consume in our diet.

Secondary bile acids are not produced in our liver. They are produced by our intestinal bacteria (this will be covered in greater detail when I discuss the microbiome). Our bile is made up of many components, all of which play a key role in creating and maintaining healthy bile. Why is this so important? The bottom line is the amount of healthy bile our liver produces daily is directly proportional to how well our body absorbs key nutrients from our diet and how well our body eliminates excess cholesterol, hormones, and other toxins from our body.

Bile is produced in our liver by hepatocytes, is stored in our gallbladder, and becomes concentrated over time. On average, our body produces nearly a liter of bile per day. Our bile performs several different functions. Its primary function is aiding the body in its digestion and absorption of fats consumed through our daily diet. Key nutrients, such as fat-soluble vitamins A, E, D, and K, and other essential fatty acids, such as alpha-linolenic acid (an omega-3 fatty acid) and linoleic acid (an omega-6 fatty acid), require bile for absorption. Thus, bile insufficiency may lead to malabsorption of fats as well as deficiencies in these essential nutrients.

When we eat, particularly a meal containing fat, two things occur:

1. *Cholecystokinin* (CCK), a peptide hormone produced in our small intestine, stimulates our pancreas to release digestive enzymes and our gallbladder to contract. This releases concentrated bile into our common bile duct.

2. The bile produced in our liver is temporarily shunted away from storage to aid digestion. The liver bile, a less concentrated bile, flows through the hepatic ducts into the common bile duct where it's joined by concentrated bile, which was expelled from the gallbladder in response to eating. Together, the concentrated bile from the gallbladder and the less concentrated bile from the liver empty directly into the upper portion of our small intestine, known as the *duodenum*, through the opening, known as the *ampulla of Vater*. More commonly, it's called the *sphincter of Oddi*. (See Image #3.)

Diagram of Liver, Pancreas, and Gallbladder

Liver

Right
hepatic duct

Common
hepatic duct

Gall bladder

Common
bile duct

Duodenum
(Intestine)

Left hepatic duct

Cystic duct

Pancreas

Pancreatic duct

Ampulla of Vater
Sphincter of Oddi

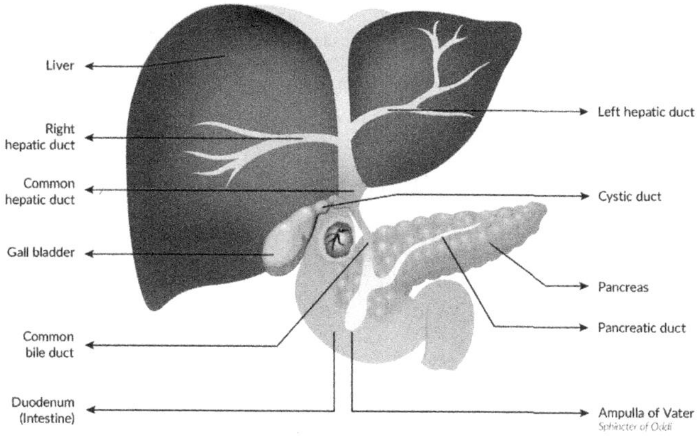

Image #3 – Diagram of Liver, Pancreas, and Gallbladder

It is here, in our duodenum, where the process of fat digestion and absorption begins. When both the liver and gallbladder are functioning properly, this process runs efficiently. However, if the bile duct is obstructed by gallstones, or if the bile is too thick or sticky to flow smoothly through the ducts, or if the gallbladder was removed, there is no longer access to stored concentrated bile.

Instead, you'll rely solely on the less concentrated bile made within your liver. We no longer have the timed release of concentrated bile triggered by eating. Over time, this leads to bile insufficiency, perpetuating further malabsorption of fats and fat-soluble nutrients and directly contributing to the onset of additional digestive challenges.

A second important function of bile is the role it plays in supporting and maintaining the pH balance within our gut. Our stomach acid pH is usually in the range of one to three on a scale of zero to fourteen (zero being the most acidic, fourteen being the least acidic), yet it reaches a pH somewhere in the neighborhood of four or five after eating.

As the contents exit the stomach and enter the first portion of the small intestine (the duodenum), the acidic contents are immediately neutralized by our bile to a pH of six to seven.[26] Aside from neutralizing the gastric secretions in the duodenum, our bile acids also play a pivotal role in maintaining the intestinal pH throughout our intestinal tract. An adequate pH is critical for the survival of healthy intestinal flora, known as the *gut microbiome*, and for sustaining the integrity of the cells lining our gut, the *enterocytes*, thus preventing inflammation and leaky gut.

In addition to supporting intestinal pH balance, a third and critical function of bile is preventing small intestinal bacterial overgrowth. Bile has potent antimicrobial properties. Think of bile, along with our other digestive enzymes, as our body's naturally produced antibiotic, antiviral, and antifungal agents for our gut. Healthy bile production and flow inhibits the overgrowth, colonization, and translocation of pathogenic microorganisms within our intestine. Therefore, anything that hinders or dampens our body's ability to produce or secrete bile will likely result in gut dysbiosis, leading to conditions such as *small intestinal bacterial overgrowth* (SIBO), *intestinal methanogen overgrowth* (IMO), or fungal overgrowth over time.

If supporting fat and nutrient absorption, neutralizing acidity to maintain intestinal pH, and killing off potential pathogens within the gut are not enough, bile also plays an imperative role in waste removal. This includes estrogens. Believe it or not, bile is one of our body's most critical absorbers and carriers of waste. All our body's cholesterol, hormones, metabolic waste, and toxicants (like carcinogens, xenobiotic chemicals, pharmaceuticals, and heavy metals such as mercury, aluminum, and lead) are filtered through and packaged up in our liver during the two phases of liver detoxification. All this waste is then secreted into our bile for transport.

Our bile delivers and empties these waste products, hormones, and toxicants into our small intestine via the sphincter of Oddi, where they are eventually excreted out of our body through our stool and urine. This is just another good reason to stay hydrated and make sure you are having healthy bowel movements each and every day to maximize elimination. The removal of these waste materials and toxicants through the intestine is referred to as *Phase 3 detoxification*. Stay tuned—I'll go into greater detail about Phase 3 detoxification and the gut microbiome in Chapter 5.

As you can see, the functions of bile are absolutely critical to our overall gut health, detoxification, and hormone balance. So much so that our body goes to great lengths to recycle as much of our bile as possible. From an energy standpoint, the production of bile is an expensive process for our body to undertake.

In its attempt to conserve energy expenditure, our body recycles up to 95 percent of our bile along its journey through our digestive tract. Amazingly, bile is not recycled just once or twice, but anywhere between four to twelve times in a given day. A majority of the recycling occurs in the distal small intestine, known as the *terminal ilium*. Some is recycled by the cells lining our bile ducts, and the small amount that escapes into our circulation is reabsorbed by the kidneys and sent back to the liver through the portal vein. This process of recycling is known as *enterohepatic circulation*.[27]

Although this recycling process is ideal for necessary items like bile or bilirubin, problems arise when items needing to be eliminated through our bowel, such as cholesterol, hormones, and other toxicants, are inadvertently recycled through our enterohepatic circulation. The inadvertent recycling of waste occurs when our bile becomes stagnant or is insufficient. Other factors, such as an impaired or disrupted gut microbiome, an inflamed or leaky gut, chronic constipation, or a diet too low in fiber, may also contribute to the inappropriate recycling of hormones, waste, and toxicants.

As a result of impaired enterohepatic recirculation, a vicious cycle of estrogen dominance and other hormonal imbalances along with elevated cholesterol and further toxicity occurs, all of which further perpetuate inflammation. And, as discussed before, inflammation is known to negatively impact our genes, predisposing us to the onset of chronic diseases.

In medical school, I was taught a trick for remembering *The Four Fs* of gallbladder disease:

- Female
- Fertile
- Fat
- Forty

These were the criteria used to describe patients most likely to present with gallbladder issues. I must admit this has proven to be true clinically, but I want to add that I am now seeing many women much younger than forty with gallbladder issues. The question is, why?

Why are women three times more likely to have gallbladder issues (e.g., stones requiring intervention, like a cholecystectomy) compared to men? Interestingly enough, research shows that our hormone levels may play a large part. As it turns out, higher levels of estrogen contribute to the formation of gallstones. As discussed in Chapter 1, during the perimenopausal years (typically this is mid-to-late thirties through our forties), estrogen dominance notoriously occurs as a woman's natural production of progesterone declines at a much faster rate than her estrogen.

What does estrogen have to do with gallstones? Estrogen enhances the action of an enzyme in our liver known as the *3-hydroxy-3-*

methylglutaryl coenzyme A (or the HMG-CoA enzyme). This enzyme is responsible for the biosynthesis of cholesterol in our liver. The higher the level of estrogen, the more action this enzyme gets to see, and the more cholesterol is produced in the liver. Higher cholesterol eventually saturates the bile, causing it to become more congested or thickened, contributing to cholesterol crystallization and gallstone formation.

Thickened bile, often referred to as bile sludge, is much harder to move out of the gallbladder and does not flow as smoothly through the bile ducts. The stagnant bile predisposes women to gallstone formation, which can further obstruct bile flow and lead to symptoms of gallbladder dysfunction and bile insufficiency.

Unfortunately, conventional treatment for most women experiencing gallbladder symptoms or dysfunction is to undergo a cholecystectomy. In some cases, this procedure may be medically necessary if the situation is life threatening, yet in a majority of cases, it's *not* life threatening. The procedure is still carried out in an attempt to alleviate symptoms. Remember—some 40 percent of patients undergoing gallbladder removal still experience long-term abdominal symptoms post removal. This is a condition known as *Postcholecystectomy Syndrome.*

We need to think twice before gallbladder removal, as it is often not the best solution. In fact, gallbladder removal will likely further perpetuate the problem of impaired estrogen metabolism. Without a gallbladder, our bile concentration and the timely secretion of bile is altered. Our elimination of estrogens, cholesterol, and other toxicants through the bile becomes further compromised. Our intestinal pH becomes distorted, negatively impacting the diversity and integrity of our gut microbiome.

An impaired gut microbiome cannot efficiently eliminate estrogen through the bowel. Instead, more estrogen is recycled via enterohepatic circulation, which further perpetuates estrogen dominance. We need to focus on preserving our gallbladder and preventing gallbladder disease. We need to focus on restoring liver function and enhancing bile flow. We need to focus on dietary and lifestyle behaviors to reduce the toxicity of our bile and enhance the production and secretion of healthy bile within our liver. This aids in maximizing the health and diversity of our gut microbiome, preventing the enterohepatic recirculation of our hormones and toxicants, thus decreasing the likelihood of hormone imbalance and disease.

Keep in mind, the health of our bile impacts the health of our hormones. The amount of healthy bile produced by our liver daily is directly proportional to the amount of hormone and toxicants we can eliminate from our body on a daily basis.

Building healthy bile matters.

IN SUMMARY

In this chapter, I discuss the five primary functions of bile:

1. Emulsify and absorb fats and cholesterol

2. Absorb fat-soluble vitamins A, E, D, and K and essential fatty acids such as *alpha-linolenic* and *linoleic* acid

3. Neutralize gastric secretions and maintain intestinal pH

4. Provide natural antimicrobial properties to ward off pathogenic gut microbes

5. Bind and deliver hormones, waste, and toxicants to the small intestine for elimination

Am I at Risk for Low Bile Flow or Bile Insufficiency?

I've provided the following list to help you determine your level of bile insufficiency. You may be at higher risk for bile insufficiency if any of the following apply:

- History of cholecystectomy (gallbladder removal)

- History of gallbladder stones or inflammation

- History of rapid weight loss (may increase bile sludge and stone formation)

- History of Nonalcoholic Fatty Liver Disease (NAFLD)— significantly reduces gallbladder motility, resulting in decreased bile outflow[28]

- Elevated liver enzymes (ALT, AST, GGT), cholesterol levels, or triglycerides

- Vitamin deficiencies (especially A, E, D, and K) and essential fatty acid deficiencies

- Parasite infections (parasites may migrate up into bile ducts causing biliary obstruction)[29]

- Estrogen dominance (elevated estrogen relative to progesterone levels)

- Medications (like *Proton Pump Inhibitors*, or PPIs)—long-term use of PPIs has been shown to induce morphological changes in the bile duct, cause focal bile duct stricture formation, and contribute to bile duct obstruction, all of which are characteristics of precancerous lesions of the bile duct[30]

What Are Signs and Symptoms Associated With Impaired Gallbladder or Bile Flow?

The following list consists of both the more common and less common signs and symptoms associated with impaired gallbladder function or bile flow:

- Upper mid- or right-sided abdominal discomfort
- Less tolerance to fatty foods (abdominal pain and diarrhea)
- Gas and bloating
- Chronic nausea
- Foul-smelling flatulence
- Pale colored stool
- *Steatorrhea* (greasy or fatty stools)
- Constipation
- *Dysbiosis* (imbalanced gut microflora)
- *Gastro-Esophageal Reflux Disease* (GERD)
- Small Intestinal Bacterial Overgrowth (SIBO) or Intestinal Methanogen Overgrowth (IMO)
- Small Intestinal Fungal Overgrowth (SIFO)

- Headaches or migraine headaches
- Fatigue
- Mood swings
- Weight gain or obesity
- Dry, itchy skin
- Difficulty making decisions (this is based in Chinese medicine theory)

Are Tests Available to Evaluate Gallbladder and Bile Function?

There are many conventional tests available to aid in evaluating the health and function of your gallbladder and bile ducts, but this is not the case when it comes to evaluating the health and function of your bile. Most often when evaluating the gallbladder, a combination of both blood test and diagnostics tests are required to make an accurate diagnosis.

Below, I have included many of the most common conventional tests used today. Unfortunately, when it comes to evaluating the health of bile, testing is much more limited. For this reason, obtaining a complete history, timeline of events, and a physical exam are critical steps to evaluating for bile insufficiency or toxic bile—something that is often overlooked in conventional medicine.

Blood Tests

A test of your complete blood count (CBC) can reveal an elevation in white blood cell count (WBC) when there is a gallbladder infection. You can also test for other things. If certain liver enzymes, like *alanine aminotransferase* (ALT), *aspartate aminotransferase* (AST), or *gamma-glutamyl transferase* (GGT) are elevated, it may indicate biliary obstruction. If there are elevated levels of bilirubin, it may be a result of gallstones limiting excretion.

Diagnostic Imaging Tests

Below is a list of other types of tests:

1. **Ultrasound**: The most commonly used imaging test determines the presence and size of gallstones, but it provides little information on the level of inflammation.

2. **X-rays**: This may detect some calcium-rich gallstones, but it cannot detect all types of stones or bile sludge.

3. **Computed tomography (CT)**: This test can be useful for detecting an infected or ruptured gallbladder, but it may not detect gallstones.

4. **Magnetic resonance imaging (MRI)**: An MRI can detect stones within the bile ducts, but it might miss infections.

5. **Endoscopic retrograde cholangiopancreatography (ERCP)**: Considered the "gold standard" test to diagnose and remove stones blocking bile ducts, complications can arise in up to 10 percent of those treated.

6. **Hepatobiliary iminodiacetic acid (HIDA) scan**: This test evaluates acute gallbladder inflammation and bile duct obstruction and measures how efficiently your gallbladder is releasing bile. It's sometimes known as *gallbladder ejection fraction*.

When it comes to gallbladder symptoms, all too often conventional medicine's answer is surgical removal. This can lead to a host of potential long-term complications. Unless the gallbladder is severely infected or the bile duct is obstructed (and removal is necessary), there are several dietary and lifestyle interventions, along with some supplementation that can support gallbladder function and help you build healthy bile.

You may have heard of a *gallbladder flush*. This is a home remedy used by many people to *cleanse* their gallbladder and *eliminate gallstones*. This is not a home remedy I recommend unless you are working with a naturopathic doctor. Clinically, I have seen side effects like nausea, vomiting, and abdominal pain in patients attempting a gallbladder flush. There is also the risk of a gallstone lodging in and blocking the bile duct.

Keep in mind, whether you're dealing with toxic bile, bile sludge, or gallstones, understand these are all symptoms of impaired function. Our goal is always to treat the cause, not the symptom. Although a gallbladder flush may sound like a good idea, it is treating the symptom. Focusing on building healthy bile, facilitating bile flow, and supporting gallbladder function are the goals. In Chapter 8, you'll learn "Seven Ways to Build Your Bile."

Chapter 4

Your Liver—The Body's Major Detoxification Organ

Patient Case Study: "Therese"

Therese is one of the most medically complex women I have had the pleasure to work with. I first met Therese, who was forty years old at the time, in July of 2019. She came to see me for her digestive challenges (frequent nausea and GERD), mood disturbances (severe anxiety), PMS with very painful periods, frequent headaches, joint and muscle pain, and episodic tingling and numbness. And, to make matters worse, she had recently experienced a miscarriage.

She admitted to experiencing very high levels of stress due to her ongoing health issues, relationship stress, financial concerns, and, eventually, the challenges brought by the COVID-19 pandemic. She was teaching full time, and at the time of our visit, she was already taking Zoloft for her mood, Dexilant for her GERD, Xanax for her anxiety and sleep, and a thyroid medication (which we immediately titrated down and discontinued, based upon her lab results).

She already had a colonoscopy (which was normal) and an endoscopy (showing mild gastritis). Because she brought prior lab results, including her genetic report from 23andMe, we were able to review and discuss them together. I shared with Therese that her genetic report provided us an opportunity to see where she might be more vulnerable medically. I further explained that although her genes were, indeed, important, it was the environment that her genes were exposed to that was most important.

Her StrateGene *report revealed SNPs in several key genes: MTHFR, COMT, PEMT, and GSTP. This helped shed light on the array of her presenting symptoms. Her MTHFR 677 gene was* Heterozygous *(+/-), meaning she was likely only methylating, a critical pathway for detoxification and antioxidant production, at about 50 percent. Her COMT gene was* Homozygous *(+/+), meaning her ability to clear out estrogen metabolites as well as break down* catecholamines (dopamine, epinephrine, norepinephrine, *and* adrenalin) *was slow.*

Additionally, she was homozygous, resulting in diminished activity for both her PEMT (the gene responsible for making phosphatidylcholine, *a critical part of cell membrane integrity and bile production), and GSTP (the genes responsible for helping her body use its primary antioxidant,* glutathione*). Our treatment approach was to first address her digestive complaints, as her gut inflammation was likely exacerbating all of her symptoms, hindering her nutritional status and further compromising her Phase 1, 2, 2.5, and 3 detoxification pathways.*

I ordered an Organic Acids Test (OAT), a urine test to evaluate intestinal microbial overgrowth (yeast, fungal, and bacterial metabolites), mitochondrial markers (how well energy is being produced), neurotransmitter metabolites, nutritional markers [levels of B12, B9 (folate), B7 (Biotin), B6, B5, B2, CoQ10, vitamin C, and NAC], and indicators for detoxification (glutathione, methylation, and toxin exposure).

While waiting for her lab results, I suggested she avoid eating out (she was doing so two to three times a week) and eliminate all processed foods, gluten, dairy, and sugar (she drank soda daily in attempts to sooth her stomach), as they were all inflammatory and might worsen her GERD symptoms. We added in supplementation of L-glutamine to soothe and support her gut, a digestive enzyme with ox bile for PEMT support and fat absorption, a binding agent to absorb intestinal toxins, and we continued her probiotics. Methylated B vitamins and magnesium for MTHFR and COMT support were also added to soothe anxiety and to promote methylation and hormone balance.

She admitted to being very sensitive to supplements and medications overall (commonly seen in individuals with methylation and detoxification challenges), so we decided to add them in one at a time. Therese decided to move forward with a GI MAP stool test, as well, to evaluate her microbiome. Her Organic Acids Test (OAT) revealed elevated levels of both yeast and Clostridia bacterial markers (major triggers for inflammation compromising overall gut health and detoxification), an altered neurotransmitter balance between dopamine and epinephrine/nor-epinephrine metabolites (likely contributing to her worsening anxiety symptoms), a significant deficiency in vitamin B12 (slowing MTHFR and detoxification), and low levels of glutathione (our body's primary antioxidant, particularly important for neutralizing estrogen metabolites).

Her GI MAP test revealed high levels of dysbiotic gut flora along with low levels of good, healthy gut flora (Bacteroidetes), *low levels of Secretory IgA (an immune response marker), and a very high level of the Beta-Glucuronidase (an enzyme produced in the microbiome, which, in high levels, potentiates estrogen recycling, contributing to estrogen dominance).*

Over the course of the next six months, treatment was difficult for Therese. She was very sensitive to the antimicrobial agents, as well as to the higher doses of methylated B vitamins, so we had to progress slowly with her treatment. She had intermittent nausea at times, making it difficult for her to comply with dietary and supplement recommendations. Her episodes of anxiety also impacted her ability to follow through. What worked best was to have weekly check-ins to help her stay on track, moving one step at time.

We worked toward establishing a more consistent sleep-wake cycle to support her energy and stress tolerance, and an eating schedule to support her blood sugar and hormone balance. Daily walks, along with Epsom salt baths, were added to support relaxation. Castor oil packs were incorporated to support her gallbladder and liver function. Herbal teas were added to sooth and support digestion and liver detoxification. Adrenal support was also added to aid in balancing her stress response.

By providing Therese with a lot of patience, frequent reassurance, and support, she began to feel safe and more confident, allowing her healing to begin. Once we were able to resolve her GERD with diet changes, bile support, and dysbiosis correction with antimicrobial herbs and probiotics (as seen on her follow-up testing), we were able to add in additional liver support to address her estrogen dominate state. She added more cruciferous vegetables and leafy greens into her diet, along with a supplement of DIM to support Phase 1 estrogen metabolism. A supplementation of liposomal glutathione was slowly added to replenish her low levels of the antioxidant necessary to support Phase 2 estrogen metabolism. Lastly, she took a supplement of calcium-D glucarate (to support lowering the high beta-glucuronidase activity in her microbiome and support Phase 3 estrogen metabolism)

Over the next two months, her PMS symptoms and headaches improved, and her DUTCH hormone testing revealed a much healthier estrogen and progesterone balance, yet she was still not methylating efficiently, as indicated by higher levels of both 2-OH and 4-OH estrogen metabolites and low levels of B12 on her lab report. Because she was so sensitive to higher oral doses of both the methylcobalamin and hydroxycobalamin forms of B12, we decided to switch over to a topical cream of methyl B12, folate, and B6 to support her methylation and replenish her low B12.

In cases such as Therese's, it is always best to start low and go slow with dosing. It is also important to remember that sometimes less is more. Taking a bunch of supplements to treat symptoms is not a good approach. Genetic and Functional laboratory testing allowed us to detect her key areas of imbalance and vulnerabilities and allowed for targeted treatment to replenish deficiencies, remove toxicities, and restore overall gut health and hormone balance. We certainly did not change Therese's genes, but we did significantly modify her diet and lifestyle, as well as add in stress reduction techniques and self-care practices to support her genes, restore her digestion, balance her hormones, and improve her overall quality of life.

Why Is the Liver So Important?

When we think of our liver, most of us think of it as being our body's filtering organ for purifying our blood. It is true that the primary role of our liver is to filter the blood before it is distributed throughout the rest of our body. What you may not be aware of are all the other vital life functions our livers perform in order to maintain our health. Some of these essential functions include:

- Producing and secreting bile to aid in digestion and absorption of fats and fat-soluble vitamins

- Metabolizing and excreting toxicants like xenoestrogens, alcohol, or medications

- Packaging and ridding our body of excess hormones, cholesterol, and bilirubin

- Storage of key nutrients, such vitamins, minerals, and glycogen (a stored form of glucose)

- Synthesizing proteins and clotting factors

- Regulating our immune response

- Activating enzymes, allowing our body to carry out thousands of additional functions every day

As you can see, our liver is much more than just a filtering organ. It is one of the most metabolically active organs in our body. Since it is such a highly metabolic organ and involved in so many different processes, it is routinely exposed to a number of insults and is highly susceptible to injury.

The good news is that our liver has an incredible ability to rapidly repair and regenerate itself. However, despite having the ability to regenerate quickly, when our liver receives insults too frequently and too repetitively, as seen in cases of chronic alcohol ingestion or living in a toxic environment, or in such a high amount as may be seen in cases of medication overdose (e.g., Tylenol), our liver becomes overwhelmed. An overwhelmed liver begins to fail in maintaining and carrying out all its vital functions, resulting in complications that can include death.

How Healthy Is My Liver?

Living in today's world, the level of environmental toxicants poses a tremendous threat to our overall health. We are exposed daily to a significantly higher level of environmental toxicants than ever before. These toxicants are entering our bodies at a rate faster than our bodies can effectively manage and remove them, resulting in the bioaccumulation, or build up, of toxicants within our body. Over time, this toxicant load places an enormous burden on our body's detoxification organs. Your liver is the primary detoxification organ, and this buildup of toxicants hinders its ability to effectively carry out its functions.

How do you know if your liver is over-burdened? Start by taking a good look at your environment and by listening to what your body is telling you. I would venture to say all of us are experiencing some of level of liver burden, some more than others. To quote one of my mentors, the late Dr. Walter Crinnion, "In today's world, if you are eating, drinking or breathing, then you are toxic."[31]

Unfortunately, today's conventional medicine and standard laboratory testing are inefficient and ineffective at detecting a burdened liver. Why? Standard laboratory testing evaluates the levels of liver enzymes (ALT, AST) in our blood to assess the structural damage to our liver cells. These tests are not assessing for how well our liver cells are functioning or how much of a burden our liver may be under.

A clinical evaluation offers the information truly needed to evaluate for liver burden. Listening to patients, taking a detailed history and timeline of events, evaluating their symptoms, and performing a physical exam provide a means to understanding the person as a whole.

This is a more beneficial way of determining the level of liver burden. Functional medicine testing is also useful, as these tests provide a deeper look into you as an individual. Early detection of liver burden allows for early intervention preserving our liver cell function. The challenge is that symptoms of liver burden, or congestion, are often initially vague and, for that reason, they are often overlooked in conventional medicine.

My patients with liver congestion commonly report many of the following symptoms:

- Generalized fatigue
- Headaches, vision changes
- Digestive changes (constipation or not emptying well)
- Fullness or distention (particularly in the upper right abdomen)
- Difficulty thinking clearly, memory decline
- Sleep disturbances (especially between one and three in the morning)
- Emotional irritability
- Skin changes (discoloration, spots, rashes, or itchiness)
- Menstrual cycle changes (for those still menstruating)
- Difficulty maintaining weight

Conventional medicine would likely treat these symptoms individually, rather than as a whole. Treatments would most likely consist of medications—pain medication for the headaches, laxatives for constipation, sleeping pills for sleep, and birth control pills for the cycle and mood issues. The problem with this approach is that only the symptoms are being addressed and not the cause. Such treatments simply add to further liver burden.

In clinical practice, I strive to treat each patient as a whole person and seek to find and address the underlying cause of their presenting symptoms. I am so grateful to have been trained in Traditional Chinese Medicine (TCM) as part of my ND training, for I often rely on my TCM training in order to find the solutions.

From a TCM perspective, the above-mentioned symptoms would result from *Liver Qi Stagnation*, or the inability of the liver energy (*Qi*) to flow as easily and freely as it should, resulting in symptoms of fatigue, abdominal fullness, ineffectual bowel elimination, menstrual cycle changes, and weight challenges. Left untreated, it will progress to *Liver Fire Rising*, resulting in symptoms like headaches, vision changes, emotional irritability, cognition challenges, and sleep disturbances.

Sleep disturbance is a common symptom. Many patients in my clinical practice report that they routinely wake up between one and three in the morning with difficulty getting back to sleep. According to the TCM body clock, the time period between one and three in the morning is associated with the liver; thus, disturbed sleep during this time is often associated with impaired liver function.

Chinese Medicine Body Clock

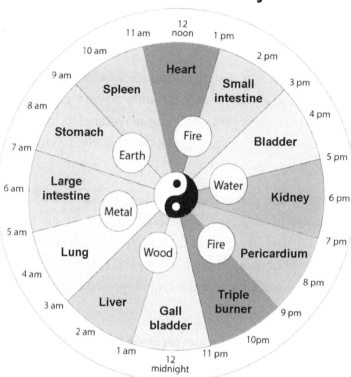

Image #4 – TCM Medicine Body Clock Wheel

This is not about treating the symptoms; it is about being able to see the bigger picture and treating the underlying cause: a stressed liver.

By treating and supporting the liver through nutrition, lifestyle interventions, specific herbs, supplements, and acupuncture, along with other detoxification practices, the symptoms begin to resolve on their own.

This is the path to true health and healing.

What Does the Liver Have to Do With Hormones?

So, why is it important to talk about the liver when discussing our hormones?

I get it. Our liver is not really considered *the sexiest* organ. So often, it's left out of the equation and certainly doesn't get the attention it deserves, especially regarding hormone balance in our body. The truth is, without healthy liver function, it is nearly impossible to have healthy hormones.

Let's start with estrogen metabolism. In Chapter 1, I addressed the silent epidemic of estrogen dominance. You may be thinking to yourself: *Where is all this estrogen coming from?* Well, most is naturally produced in your ovaries, adrenal glands, and fat cells. From the onset of menarche up until the onset of menopause, our ovaries are our primary producers of estrogen.

After menopause, our body relies on our adrenal glands and, to some extent, our fat cells for the production of estrogen. This is an important point to remember. Our adrenal glands are our body's natural backup system for menopause. They have the ability to produce sex hormones to support our body in aging healthfully during our menopausal years. However, if they become depleted by chronic stressors—potential causes being dietary, environmental, physical, or emotional—they become less efficient in supporting hormone production and balance.

Supporting and maintaining healthy adrenal gland function plays a key role in hormone balance before, during, and after our menopause years. For now, let's get back to estrogen: where it comes from and how it's metabolized.

Unfortunately, due to environmental influences, an ever-increasing amount of estrogen is coming into our bodies from exogenous sources. One source is our diet. A majority of the animal products consumed in today's American diet, unless organic, free-range, or wild-caught, are laden with hormones—along with antibiotics, pesticides, and other toxicants, which present another set of challenges for our liver and gut flora.

Hormones are used in food-producing animals to accelerate the growth rate of the animals and to enhance their yield. Faster growth and a higher yield mean higher profits in a shorter period of time. Unfortunately, these agricultural practices continue despite mounting evidence of the disastrous effects it has on the health and well-being of the animals, as well as those of us consuming them and their products.

Evidence makes it clear that the excess steroid hormones found in dairy products are an important risk factor for various cancers in humans.[32,33] Evidence also confirms that cows treated with recombinant bovine growth hormone—rBGH, a synthetic hormone made in a laboratory—to increase milk production have much higher rates of mastitis—inflammation in their udders, leading to higher concentrations of bacteria in their milk—and they are more often treated with antibiotics.[34] Therefore, consuming milk and dairy products in your daily diet, which is popularly touted as *healthy*, may be exposing you to higher levels of external hormones, bacteria, and antibiotics.

Aside from hormones, the continued use of antibiotics in food-producing animals (cattle, swine, and poultry) poses another significant health concern. It is estimated that as much as 80 percent of all antibiotics produced in the United States are used in food-producing animals.[35] And on December 10, 2019, the U.S. Food and Drug Administration released its 2018 summary report on antimicrobials sold or distributed for use in food-producing animals. It showed a 9 percent increase from 2017 to 2018.[36]

This is not the direction we should be moving in. The ongoing use of antibiotics in animals brings up an even greater risk for the development of antibiotic-resistant strains of bacteria, or *superbugs*, posing a huge threat to our long-term health. Additionally, we now know the negative effects antibiotics have on our gut microbiome.

As you can see, eating our Standard American Diet (SAD), rich in animal products, is directly contributing to our hormonal imbalance and an impaired gut microbiome. As you will see in Chapter 5, an impaired gut microbiome further perpetuates hormonal imbalance and estrogen dominance in particular.

Toxins All Around

Another factor contributing to the epidemic hormone imbalance crisis seen today is environmental toxicity. We are surrounded by xenoestrogens. When they enter our body, they not only interfere with our body's estrogen receptors, but they also disrupt our body's natural estrogen metabolism and detoxification pathways. Some of the most common sources of xenoestrogen encountered in our daily lives come from plastics, pesticides, personal care products, electronics, and exhaust fumes.

Exposure Sources Diagram

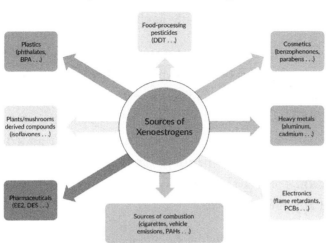

Image #5 – Exposure Sources Diagram

Once inside our body, some xenoestrogens have the ability to disrupt estrogen-signaling pathways, while others bind to estrogen receptors, stimulating the cells to respond as they do when estrogen hormone binds to them. Ultimately, all this leads to altered cell function, increased cell proliferation, and increased risk for the development of cancers.[37] Additionally, xenoestrogens clog up the natural detoxification pathways in our liver.

Our body utilizes the same liver detoxification pathways to clear out both natural estrogens and xenoestrogen. So, the higher the levels of xenoestrogens, the more overburdened our liver becomes, hindering the clearance of both natural estrogen and xenoestrogen. The end result is hormone imbalance, estrogen dominance, toxicant overload, and an increased risk for disease, especially cancer.

If that wasn't enough, xenoestrogens are also known to be fat-storing molecules. The higher the levels of xenoestrogen exposure and accumulation in our body, the more likely we are to store fat and gain weight. This may help women better understand why maintaining their weight becomes more challenging as they transition into menopause.

Every woman experiences a state of natural estrogen dominance as her progesterone levels decline faster than her estrogen levels during her perimenopause years. However, estrogen dominance becomes exacerbated when there is also a bioaccumulation of exogenous estrogens and xenoestrogens from our environment added into the mix. This leads to a competition for clearance and overburdened detoxification pathways, which is not a good combination for any woman of any age.

This may also help explain why we are seeing such an overall increase in weight gain and obesity for women of all ages. Many of these xenoestrogens are categorized as *obesogens*, meaning they induce weight gain. As you can see, the amount of external hormone exposure through foods compounded with environmental toxicant exposures is directly contributing to estrogen imbalance.

Soy and Hormones

Any discussion regarding hormone balance would not be complete without including the topic of soy. Soy fits into a category of food containing *phytoestrogens*, which are plant compounds that perform very weak estrogen-like actions in our body. Phytoestrogens are found in a variety of foods, including soybeans, tofu, flaxseeds and sesame seeds, whole grains, beans, lentils, garlic, and some fruits and vegetables. The phytoestrogens found in fruits, whole grains, and seeds are called *ligands*, while those found in soy are referred to as *isoflavones*.

The challenge with soy lies in the level of controversy surrounding its impact on our hormone health. Are phytoestrogens good for you or bad for you? That is the question.

When we think of phytoestrogens most of us think of soy—and with good reason. It's been talked about most frequently and is heavily researched. To simply make a blanket statement that soy is bad for us is not a fair statement. Unfortunately, that is what we frequently hear.

A large volume of research exists regarding the pros and cons of soy and the impact it has on cancer risk specifically. Why are the studies so conflicting? In its natural form, soy is a whole plant-based food, and research strongly shows that eating a diet rich in whole, plant-based foods has many positive effects on our body. We did not fully understand the mechanisms of how these positive effects occurred until we gained a much greater understanding of our gut microbiome. Research has confirmed that our gut microbiome can be altered by dietary interventions in ways that prevent and treat various diseases.[38]

You read that correctly: food can be our body's best medicine.

Enzymes within whole plant-based foods are able to communicate with the microorganisms in our gut. Processed foods, empty of both nutrients and enzymes, cannot communicate and may actually induce harm to our gut microbiome. The extent to which soy is processed changes the effects of its isoflavones. Breast cancer research shows that the higher the concentration of highly processed soy and soy protein isolate, the more stimulated the estrogen receptors in breast tumors; whereas the more purified diets, containing equivalent amounts soy, did not stimulate the growth of estrogen-dependent breast cancer tumors.[39]

The health and composition of your gut microbiome also matter. The potential health benefits of soy ingestion are related to how well the microbes in your colon are able to convert the soy isoflavones in their key metabolites during digestion, as different metabolites have different actions and effects.

If you choose to eat soy, consume only non-GMO (Genetically Modified Organisms) soy. Soybeans are the number-one genetically modified crop in the world. Nearly all soy—about 94 percent of soy in the United States—is genetically engineered to be herbicide tolerant (HT).[40] Research continues to reveal that the herbicides commonly used in treating these genetically modified crops—Roundup, most often—have devastating effects on our microbiome, disrupt the natural detoxification pathways, contribute to intestinal permeability, trigger inflammation, and, over time, directly contribute to a host of chronic disease.[41]

This is why I would like to rephrase the question and ask: *Is soy good for you?*

The answer: Yes, as long as it is non-GMO and unprocessed, such as edamame, homemade soy milk, or homemade tofu. Soy is a good source of dietary protein, especially for vegans and vegetarians, and it poses minimal health effects.

There is one additional piece of information worth mentioning. For those of you who are vegetarian or vegan, who may be ingesting large amounts of soy protein in your daily diet, you might be slowing down your thyroid function. Large amounts of soy isoflavones can inhibit the deiodinase enzymes in your body. These deiodinase enzymes are responsible for converting your naturally produced T4 thyroid hormone (less active) into T3 thyroid hormone (active hormone). When the body is unable to efficiently convert T4 to T3, symptoms of hypothyroid may manifest. The following case study is a good example of this:

Patient Case Study – "Carol D"

I first met Carol D. in June of 2009, a few weeks after she had been diagnosed with coronary artery disease via a Heart CT and calcium score.

She was fifty-nine, retired, and menopausal. She came to me seeking additional information and possible alternative treatment options since she had been completely asymptomatic and had been living what she called "a healthy lifestyle." She exercised five days a week and was a nonsmoker and nondrinker. She ate a vegetarian diet and was highly social with a close network of friends. However, she was concerned due to a family history of heart disease (her father passed of sudden cardiac death at age seventy-one).

She was reluctant to take the prescribed statin medication, Simvastatin (10 mg daily), because of the side effects. She had a past medical history of hypothyroidism, for which she had been taking Synthroid (50 mcg) daily for years, a mildly elevated total cholesterol and LDL cholesterol, for which she managed with diet and exercise, and had been on estrogen-only replacement therapy since 2008. Her only complaints at the time of our initial appointment were minor—a mild energy dip each afternoon and challenges with staying asleep at night.

As with all my new patients, I had her sign a records release in order to obtain her prior lab tests for review. I sent her home with a diet diary and digestive health survey. Her labs revealed high total cholesterol of 239 mg/ dL, high LDL cholesterol of 159 mg/dL, and healthy HDL at 77 mg/dL. Despite taking Synthroid, her thyroid stimulating hormone (TSH) level was borderline high at 4.14 (normal 0.4–4.50 uIU/mL with optimal being 1–2.5). There were no labs done measuring her actual thyroid hormone levels (T4 and T3).

Her diet diary revealed a high and frequent intake of goitrogenic foods— naturally occurring substances that can interfere with thyroid gland function. She had three to four servings of soy products daily, almonds as primary nut intake, and a variety of raw cruciferous vegetables daily (remember: she was a vegetarian). Based upon on her prior labs and diet diary findings, I ordered a full thyroid panel and found that her T3 level was "below normal" at 2.0 (normal 2.3–4.2 pg/mL), T4 level was normal at 1.4 (normal 0.8–1.7 ng/dL), and TSH was normal, yet not optimal, at 3.63 (optimal being 1–2.5 uIU/mL).

Despite taking her Synthroid medication daily, Carol's body was not converting her medication, which was T4, over to the active form of thyroid, which was T3. She was still in a hypothyroid state despite taking her medication, yet this fact had been missed due to incomplete lab testing and evaluation.

Long-term hypothyroidism contributes to elevated total and LDL cholesterol, atherosclerosis, and risk for coronary artery disease. I educated Carol on the relationship between her thyroid function and her heart health. I also educated her on goitrogenic foods and how, when consumed in high amounts over long periods of time, they may interfere with her thyroid T4 to T3 conversion.

I encouraged her to steam the cruciferous vegetables to decrease their goitrogenic activity to support her thyroid, vary her nut and seed intake (Brazil nuts, for example, are rich in selenium content, which is essential for thyroid function), and limit her soy intake. All would benefit her thyroid function and support T4 to T3 conversion. I also discussed other key nutrients needed for healthy T4 to T3 conversion such as iodine (commonly deficient in a vegetarian diet), selenium, and zinc. To support her nutrient levels, I also added in vitamins D3, B12, and omega-3 fatty acids (again, all these may be deficient in a vegetarian diet and are vital to cardiovascular health).

On August 24, 2009, after two months of patient education, dietary modification, and nutritional supplementation for thyroid and cholesterol, her repeated lab tests were remarkably improved with a reduction in total cholesterol (235–189 mg/dL), a reduction in LDL (145–103 mg/dL), and a reduction in THS (3.63–2.01). Her baseline Free T3 had been low at 2.0 (normal 2.3–4.2 pg/mL) and was now normal at 2.8, along with a normal T4 level at 1.1 (normal 0.8–1.7 ng/dL).

At the time of the follow-up appointment, Carol also reported an improvement in her overall sleep and fewer mid-afternoon energy dips. We discussed thyroid dosage and options for the addition of T3 or switching to a desiccated form of T4 and T3, such as Nature-Throid or compounded. She opted to continue with Synthroid, as she felt it was now working well for her. She continued her thyroid support formula, cholesterol support formula, fiber, dietary modification, and exercise routine with recommended follow-up visits every six months.

Carol's case is a great example of the power of natural medicine. Had she followed conventional medicine's recommendation, she simply would have been placed on a statin medication to treat her symptom of elevated cholesterol. Instead, she chose to seek out and treat the cause of her high cholesterol, which was determined to be hypothyroid-induced hyperlipidemia. With just a few modifications to her diet and the replenishment of key nutrients, her thyroid function was restored, and hyperlipidemia resolved. The statin medication would certainly not have been able to do that.

I feel this is important information for those of you taking thyroid (T4) replacement therapy. For those of you taking T4 medication (Synthroid, Levoxly, or levothyroxine) you may not be converting T4 to the active T3 hormone efficiently. This will cause you to continue experiencing low thyroid symptoms despite taking your medication and may contribute to other chronic conditions like elevated cholesterol, constipation, and estrogen dominance. I recommend you request a full thyroid panel to evaluate your levels—TSH, Total and Free T4, and Total and Free T3.

There are many potential causes for a reduced T4 to T3 conversion: impaired liver function, chronic stress, infections, inflammation, pesticides, heavy metals, nutritional deficiencies, and more. Be aware that a high dietary intake of soy isoflavones could be one potential cause.

Additionally, I will mention our liver and gut play key roles in our thyroid function. That's right: a majority of the T4 to T3 conversion process takes place in your liver and gut. Once again, I have to stress the importance of maintaining your liver and gut health in order to maximize the benefits of your thyroid hormone.

Estrogen, Metabolism, and the Liver

In Chapter 1, I discussed how our endogenous estrogens are produced primarily in our ovaries, adrenal glands, and fat cells. So, what happens to the hormones once they have done their job? How does our body rid itself of hormones?

In order to maintain balance, our body must be able to effectively and efficiently eliminate hormones, a process known as *estrogen metabolism*. Two key determinants for how well our body metabolizes estrogens: your nutrient status, and the health of your gut (gallbladder, liver, and microbiome). A healthy, diversified, whole-foods diet is needed to provide our bodies with a steady supply of the nutrients necessary to support estrogen metabolism and elimination. And a healthy gut allows for the absorption and assimilation of the nutrients necessary for estrogen metabolism as well as an elimination route for estrogens.

Estrogens, along with our sex and adrenal hormones (commonly referred to as steroid hormones), are synthesized from our body's cholesterol, LDL cholesterol specifically. Because they are synthesized from cholesterol, they are fat-soluble molecules rather than water soluble. This means that in order to get out of our body, the estrogens must be converted into a more water-soluble state that allows them to eventually be eliminated through the stool and urine.

To be excreted from our body, estrogens must be broken down in our liver (Phase 1), converted to more water-soluble molecules in the liver (Phase 2), transported out of the liver cells into our bile (Phase 2.5), and emptied into our intestine, where they may be further impacted by our gut microbiome. Then they are eventually eliminated through our bowel movements and urine (Phase 3). The importance of healthy bowel movements daily and staying well hydrated must not be overlooked or underestimated when it comes to maintaining hormone balance.

The complexity of estrogen metabolism can be simplified by breaking it down into three phases. Each phase requires key enzymes and specific nutrients in order to carry out its function. Although independent of each other, each phase is reliant on the others in order to effectively and efficiently metabolize and excrete estrogens. What's interesting is that research is showing us how each of these phases may be impacted by such things as dietary choices, lifestyle behaviors, environmental exposures, medications, chronic stress, and sleep cycles. Let's take a closer look at each phase.

Phase 1

If you recall from Chapter 1, there are three primary types of estrogen: estrone (E1), estradiol (E2), and estriol (E3). Think of these as the parent estrogens. During Phase 1, often referred to as the *hydroxylation* phase, E1 and E2 (along with other steroid hormones and xenobiotics) are acted upon by liver enzymes, collectively known as the *Cytochrome P450* (CYPs) system. The primary job of the CYP 450 enzymes is to change the structure of the parent estrogens by adding a hydroxyl group (-OH) to them. The addition of the hydroxyl group is what converts the parent estrogens into their more reactive intermediate metabolites.

These estrogen metabolites are often referred to as *catechol estrogen metabolites* (2-hydroxyestrone, 4-hydroxyestrone, 2-hydroxyestradiol, 4-hydroxyestradiol, and 16α-hydroxyestrone). The numbers 2, 4, or 16 correlate with the location where the hydroxyl group was attached to the parent estrogen molecule. This is important as it plays a role in determining how reactive the metabolite is within the body.

For example, the 2-OH metabolite has a weaker binding ability, and therefore is considered the safer of the estrogen metabolites. In contrast, both 4-OH and the 16-OH have a much stronger binding capacity and are more likely to stimulate tissue growth. For this reason, they are considered to be potentially more dangerous, more likely to induce DNA damage, and to contribute to a development of cancer.

The goal in Phase 1 of estrogen metabolism is to potentiate or enhance the 2-OH pathway in order to reduce the overall cancer risks. We now know that our dietary choices, lifestyle behaviors, and consumption of specific nutrients play key roles in either supporting the 2-OH pathway or inhibiting it.

What can you do to support your 2-OH pathway and decrease your potential risk? In Chapter 9, I discuss different dietary and lifestyle interventions you can make, along with nutritional supplementation to maximize your estrogen detoxification pathways.

Because these estrogen metabolites, especially 4-OH and 16-OH, are highly reactive molecules, they must be dampened to prevent damaging our DNA. The potential danger of the reactive estrogen metabolites significantly decreases once they become methylated and conjugated during Phase 2 of estrogen metabolism: detoxification.

Think of it this way: In the Phase 1 of estrogen metabolism, enzymes change the structure of the parent estrogens in an attempt to make them more recognizable by the enzymes in Phase 2. Once the Phase 2 enzymes recognize the estrogen metabolites, they can dampen their reactivity by methylating and conjugating them. This makes them more water-soluble and easier to eliminate.

The best outcome occurs when the speed of Phase 1 detoxification (parent estrogens converted into their metabolites) is equal to the speed of Phase 2 detoxification (the methylation and conjugation of the metabolites to decrease their reactivity). However, living in today's world, the balance between Phase 1 and Phase 2 activity is easily disrupted.

Environmental toxicants, chemicals, and xenoestrogens are known to induce or accelerate Phase 1 enzymes, resulting in the buildup of these highly reactive estrogen metabolites. Higher levels of reactive metabolites increase our risk for tissue damage and cancer. Despite this, there is good news. We have the ability to change this.

Research now clearly shows that both our dietary choices and lifestyle behaviors can significantly modulate estrogen metabolism. Our daily choices can shift estrogen metabolism toward the less harmful 2-OH pathway in Phase 1 as well as enhance the enzymes of the Phase 2 pathways, preventing the back up of reactive metabolites, thus decreasing our risk.[42]

One important point to mention regarding our CYP 450 Phase 1 enzymes: they are *heme* dependent, meaning they require a steady supply of iron in order to function properly. Therefore, if you are iron deficient or anemic, it may negatively impact your body's ability to metabolism estrogen, xenoestrogens, and other toxicants.

There are a few common causes of low-iron or anemic states. Menstruating women are more likely to experience lower iron or anemic states simply due to monthly bleeding cycles, particularly if cycles are long, heavy, or occurring too frequently, sooner than every twenty-eight days. Experiencing long, heavy, or frequent cycles may be a symptom of preexisting estrogen dominance. Strict vegetarian or vegan diets may also pose a potential risk for low iron or anemic states in women of any age. And *hypochlorhydria*, or low production of stomach acid, hinders our ability to extract and absorb the iron in our food.

Okay. I know what you just read may have been a bit more technical than you may have liked, so here's the "Cliff Notes" version:

- Phase 1 estrogen detoxification is a process in which our cytochrome P450 supergene family of enzymes chemically transform our fat-soluble parent estrogens into reactive intermediate metabolites. Why? So they can eventually be recognized and made water soluble by our Phase 2 enzymes.

- There are three potential estrogen metabolites: 2, 4, and 16 hydroxy estrogens. The 2 hydroxy is considered the safer estrogen metabolite, as it is the least reactive. The 4 and the 16 hydroxy estrogens can be damaging to our DNA and increase our risk for cancer if they are not neutralized by our Phase 2 enzymes.

- Our goal with estrogen detoxification is to support our body through dietary and lifestyle choices that potentiate the 2-hydroxy pathway and balance the speed of enzyme activity between Phases 1 and 2 detoxification.

- How can you modify your diet and lifestyle choices to support your estrogen metabolism? *Chapter 9: Love Your Liver* will outline this information for you.

Phase 2

Now that our parent estrogens, E1, E2, and E3, have been converted into catechol estrogen metabolites by the CYP 450 enzymes during Phase 1, they are recognizable and acted upon by the enzymes in Phase 2 detoxification. This phase encompasses two processes: methylation and conjugation.

The process of methylation is carried out by the *catechol-O-methyltransferase* (COMT) enzyme, whereby the enzyme's job is to attach a methyl group (CH3) to the catechol estrogen metabolites, rendering them less reactive and toxic in the body. The process of conjugation is carried out by additional Phase 2 enzymes, *UDP-glucuronosyltransferases,* *glutathione-S-transferase* *(GST),* and *sulfotransferases.* The conjugation of estrogens with glucuronic acid and sulfate results in the formation of water-soluble metabolites, which are then packaged in our liver and made ready for transport into our intestine and kidneys for elimination.

Methylation

To methylate our estrogen metabolites and render them less reactive, our body needs to have healthy, functioning COMT enzymes. For the COMT enzymes to function, they need a steady supply of two specific co-factors: magnesium and *S-adenosyl-methionine* (SAM). Deficiencies in either co-factor can result in slower COMT enzyme activity and thus alter estrogen metabolism.

Magnesium is one of the most critical nutrients for our body. This one mineral is involved in over 300 different enzyme systems in our body. Thus, a magnesium deficiency can lead to a host of health issues far beyond impaired estrogen metabolism.

Attempting to consume adequate amounts of magnesium in our daily diet alone is challenging. Many factors can, and do, interfere. They range from our dietary choices to the medications we take, our chronic stress levels, our gut health, and alcohol consumption. Although I always attempt to use food first, I find in clinical practice that supplementation with a good quality magnesium is often needed for my patients to get a sufficient amount.

Table 2: Selected Food Sources of Magnesium[43]

Food	Serving Size	Milligrams (mg) per serving	Percent DV*
Pumpkin seeds, roasted	1 oz	156	37
Chia seeds	1 oz	111	26
Almonds, dry roasted	1 oz	80	19
Spinach, boiled	½ cup	78	19
Cashews, dry roasted	1 oz	74	18
Peanuts, oil roasted	¼ cup	63	15
Cereal, shredded wheat	2 lg biscuits	61	15
Soymilk, plain or vanilla	1 cup	61	15
Black beans, cooked	½ cup	60	14
Edamame, shelled, cooked	½ cup	50	12
Peanut butter, smooth	2 tbs	49	12
Potato, baked with skin	3.5 oz	43	10
Rice, brown, cooked	½ cup	42	10
Yogurt, plain, low fat	8 oz	42	10
Breakfast cereals, fortified	1 serving	42	10
Oatmeal, instant	1 packet	36	9
Kidney beans, canned	½ cup	35	8
Banana	1 medium	32	8
Salmon, Atlantic, cooked	3 oz	26	6
Milk	1 cup	24–27	6
Halibut, cooked	3 oz	24	6
Raisins	½ cup	23	5
Bread, whole wheat	1 slice	23	5
Avocado, cubed	½ cup	22	5
Chicken breast, roasted	3 oz	22	5
Beef, ground, 90% lean	3 oz	20	5
Broccoli, chopped, cooked	½ cup	12	3
Rice, white, cooked	½ cup	10	2
Apple	1 medium	9	2
Carrot, raw	1 medium	7	2

*DV = Daily Value as developed by the
U.S. Food and Drug Administration (FDA)*

Unlike magnesium, SAM can be synthesized in our body through what is known as the *methylation cycle*, just as long as the methylation cycle has a steady supply of the key nutrients it requires to function. These nutrients include vitamins B2, B6, B12, and folate, along with choline, *trimethylglycine* (TMG), and methionine.

Are you beginning to see the critical role nutrients play in our body? Nutrient deficiencies directly affect enzyme function which, in turn, directly impacts how well our body can function. Unfortunately, Western medicine does not adequately address the importance of nutrients. It is for this reason that I feel compelled to include a few vital statistics here for you.

The 2015–2020 Dietary Guidelines state that magnesium intake in the United States is insufficient.[44] And, according to the recent U.S. national survey, NHANES 2007–2010 Dietary Survey, more than half of the United States population (ages four years and older) have intakes below the Estimated Average Requirement (EAR) for magnesium.[45]

This is a *huge* public health concern, yet it gets very little attention in mainstream medicine. If you recall, I mentioned that there are over 300 enzyme systems in our body reliant upon magnesium to function. Why, then, are we experiencing such a magnesium deficiency? There are many reasons, but I'm going to focus on the three I continuously see in clinical practice:

- Dietary choices—we are simply not getting what we need from our diets.

- Overall stress level—we lose magnesium through our urine when we are stressed.

- Frequent use of medications (PPIs, specifically)—inhibit our ability to absorb magnesium from foods or supplements.

Of course, there are factors other than nutrient deficiencies that impact enzyme function. However, I primarily focus on the nutrient deficiency because this is one area we can significantly change if we choose to. What we eat and drink, think, and do in our daily lives truly matters.

The COMT enzyme deserves some additional attention. Not only does the COMT enzyme support our body with estrogen detoxification, but also it supports our body with the breakdown of our catecholamine neurotransmitters: dopamine, epinephrine, and norepinephrine (commonly known as adrenalin).

Hormones and neurotransmitters are uniquely connected by the same enzyme. COMT works to aid our body in clearing out both our estrogen and neurotransmitters. So, what happens if our COMT enzyme is not functioning efficiently? Well, that depends upon whether the COMT enzyme activity is normal, fast, or slow.

This is where our genetics come into play. Some people are born with specific gene mutations or *single nucleic polymorphisms* (SNPs). Each SNP represents a difference in a single DNA building block. Most SNPs have very little, if any, effect on our overall health and development because they are located in areas of our DNA that do not impact the actual structure or function of the gene. However, in cases where the SNP occurs within our gene and impacts the structure, such as within the COMT gene, it may affect how that gene functions.

Notice I wrote that it *may affect* how that gene functions. This is an important point. Just because someone is born with a genetic SNP does not necessarily mean that person has a problem. It simply means the function of that gene may be impacted if the demands placed upon that gene are too high for too long.

For example, let's say you have been under a great deal of stress, not sleeping well, and reaching for sugar, carbohydrates, or caffeine to keep going. You're eating on the run, possibly drinking alcohol in the evening to calm down, and because you are feeling fatigued you are not getting any exercise. Do you think these behaviors disrupt your genes?

Absolutely they do!

The longer the gene, whether it has an SNP or not, is placed in this situation or similar situations, the more likely something is going to go wrong, and the gene is more likely to malfunction.

This is the point I want to drive home: the environment our genes are put into is a determining factor in our health.

What an SNP truly represents is an area of potential vulnerability for that individual gene. You see, our genes are not necessarily our destiny. Our genes are influenced heavily by the environment we put them into. As much as 85 percent of our genes' chance of expression, or being *turned on*, is due to our environment.

Yes, that's correct. Our genes respond to both our external and internal environments.

There is a whole field of scientific study focusing on this very topic. *Epigenetics* looks at the interaction between our genes and our environment. Epigenetics also studies how environmental factors can impact how our genes respond without changing the DNA sequencing of the gene itself.

Several lifestyle factors have been identified that impact epigenetic patterns, including:

- Diet
- Obesity
- Physical activity
- Tobacco smoking

- Alcohol consumption
- Environmental pollutants
- Psychological stress
- Sleep disturbances—working night shifts

Each of these factors have been found to impact epigenetic patterns.[46]

The good news here is that our genes' destiny is, to a large extent, in our own hands. How we choose to live our life, and what we eat, drink, think, and do have the ability to turn on or turn off our genes.

If we do have an SNP in our COMT gene, resulting in a slower COMT enzyme activity, we may be at greater risk for impaired estrogen metabolism, particularly if we are magnesium deficient or not methylating well or both. A slower COMT can lead to an increased risk for PMS symptoms, estrogen dominance, and potential cancers. Additionally, slower COMT activity can result in elevated neurotransmitter levels leading to mood challenges, anxiety, irritability, and sleep disturbances.

Since the COMT enzyme is responsible for both estrogen detoxification and neurotransmitter breakdown, any inefficiency of the enzyme, or a deficiency of its co-factors magnesium or SAM, may result in both hormonal imbalance as well neurotransmitter imbalance. Keep in mind though, even in cases where we have a completely normal functioning COMT gene and healthy COMT enzyme levels, the environment we put that gene in can overwhelm its ability to keep up with the demand, leading to the same symptoms as would present in cases of slower COMT enzyme activity.

Aside from having an SNP in the COMT Gene, other situations are also known to slow down COMT gene function. Being in an estrogen dominant state; having infections within our gut; being under prolonged periods of high stress; exposure to toxins, like bisphenols found in plastics; and the bioactive ingredients in foods, such as green tea or quercetin, can all slow down COMT activity.

Medications can also significantly impact COMT activity. There is an entire class of medications that are COMT inhibitors, specifically used as an adjunctive therapy with Carbidopa-Levodopa in the treatment of Parkinson's disease. Higher levels of serotonin have been shown to slow COMT activity.[47] This is of concern. One of six adults in the United States is taking some kind of psychiatric drug, most likely an antidepressant. Those of you taking Selective Serotonin Reuptake Inhibitor (SSRI) medications, such as Zoloft, Paxil, Prozac, Celexa, or Lexapro, please be aware the medication may be impacting your COMT activity.

As you can see, insults coming from many directions can negatively impact the function of our genes. Dr. Ben Lynch, author of *Dirty Genes*, does a great job describing in his book how our genes get dirty from our diet, lifestyle, and environment and what we can do to clean them. I highly recommend you take a look at his book for more information on the COMT gene, as well as several other medically relevant SNPs known to play a potential role in our overall physical, mental, and emotional well-being.

We have the power to prevent disease by supporting our genes. I encourage you to start by taking a closer look at yourself, your surroundings, and your lifestyle. Follow this by tuning in and listening to what these things are telling you. What can you learn about yourself?

A discussion about genetics and the role SNPs may play regarding estrogen detoxification would not be complete without addressing the methylation cycle and what is referred to as the *Methylenetetrahydrofolate reductase* (MTHFR) gene.

Together, the COMT gene and MTHFR gene play key roles in our body's metabolism of estrogens and xenoestrogens. The methylation cycle is a very complex series of pathways.

Methylation

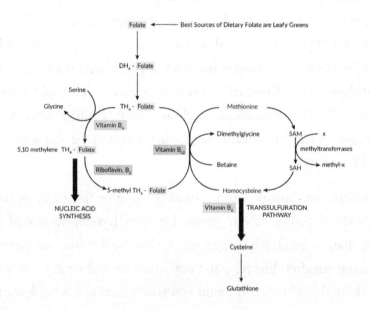

Image #6 – Methylation

The methylation cycle is made up of the folate cycle and the methionine cycle collectively. It receives a great deal of attention these days, which it deserves, as it is one of the most important metabolic pathways in our body.

Methylation significantly impacts our health by regulating several functions in the body, including:

- Genetic expression and our DNA repair processes
- Inflammatory response
- Immune response (protection against infections)

- Glutathione production and recycling (our body's most important antioxidant)
- Neurotransmitter formation and breakdown (brain chemistry)
- Mitochondrial function and energy production
- Detoxification of hormones, heavy metals, and chemicals

In order for our methylation cycle to run effectively and efficiently, and carry out these processes, a steady supply of nutrients is required. These nutrients include methylated vitamin B2, B6, B12, folate (vitamin B9), trimethylglycine (TMG), choline, and methionine.

Where do these nutrients come from? Primarily through our daily diet and possibly through supplementation. Just another reminder of how important nutrition and digestive health are to our body's ability to function. Deficiencies in any of these nutrients, especially folate and vitamin B12, will negatively impact our body's methylation cycle. Unfortunately, such deficiencies are quite common today.

Diets higher in processed food are depleted of nutrients and often high in synthetic materials, folic acid being one. I stress this point because folic acid and folate are not the same thing, nor do they work the same way in our body. Naturally occurring folate comes from real food, dark leafy greens topping the list, whereas folic acid, a synthetically made vitamin, is added to processed and prepackaged foods such as breads, cereals, and crackers. Labels on food items stating "fortified" or "enriched" most often contain added folic acid.

Lesser quality multivitamins and supplements will also include folic acid, not folate, as an ingredient. Reading labels is important. Why is this a problem? Well, many of us are getting too little folate and too much folic acid in our daily diet. These higher levels of folic acid can compete with folate and slow down our body's methylation cycle.

For individuals who have an SNP in their MTHFR gene, this can pose even more of a concern. Individuals with a genetic SNP in their

MTHFR gene have a decreased ability to convert folic acid to folate from the start. Therefore, diets high in folic acid may result in a buildup of folic acid and a deficiency of the much-needed folate. Over time, this poses a greater health risk, as high levels of unmethylated folic acid have been shown to not only slow down our methylation cycle, but also may contribute to an increased risk of cancer.

Another cause of nutritional deficiencies stems from eating highly restrictive diets over long periods of time. Individuals living a strict vegetarian or vegan lifestyle may run a higher risk of vitamin B12 deficiency, since B12 is found almost exclusively in meat. I am an advocate for eating a plant-based diet, but I want to stress the importance of doing so appropriately, by supplementing vitamin B12.

Vitamin B12 deficiency is a health concern. Vegetarians and vegans are often found to be vitamin B12 deficient. One does not have to be vegan or vegetarian to become B12 deficient. Even those of us consuming animal products in our diet can have difficulty absorbing the B12 from our food if our natural production of hydrochloric acid (HCL) or pancreatic enzymes is too low. Because our natural production of both declines with age, we are more susceptible to B12 deficiency as we age.

Other factors that may contribute to altered B12 absorption include preexisting medical conditions, such as:

- Pernicious anemia
- Crohn's disease
- Celiac disease
- Helicobacter pylori infection
- Small intestinal bacterial overgrowth (SIBO)
- Parasitic infections

All these conditions have been shown to impact B12 absorption. Prior surgical procedures, such partial gastrectomy or gastric bypass surgery, typically result in decreased B12 absorption. Both prescription and over-the-counter medications, like antibiotics, metformin, PPIs, histamine blockers, and nonsteroidal anti-inflammatory drugs (NSAIDs), are a significant, and often overlooked, cause of altered B12 absorption.

Why are methylfolate and B12 so important? Think of it this way: methylfolate and B12 are the dynamic duo keeping the gears of both the folate and the methionine cycles turning. When deficient, the methionine cycle slows and the natural synthesis of SAM, our body's primary methyl donor, declines. If you recall, SAM is one of the primary cofactors necessary for our COMT enzyme function. And our COMT enzyme function is one of the regulators of our estrogen metabolism.

With a healthy, functioning MTHFR gene and a steady supply of cofactors, the gears of both the folate and the methionine cycles keep on turning, resulting in a steady synthesis of SAM. With a steady supply of SAM, along with magnesium, our COMT enzyme is able to carry out its function to efficiently metabolize estrogen. If we have an SNP in the MTHFR gene, our body's ability to convert folate into its active state (*5-methyltetrathydrofolate* or methylfolate), may be slowed. The degree to which it is slowed is variable, ranging from 30–80 percent, depending upon the specifics of the SNP.[48] Therefore, having an SNP in our MTHFR gene can lead to low methylfolate levels.

Low methylfolate levels can lead to a slowed methylation cycle overall and can lead to a lower natural production of SAM, which can then lead to altered COMT enzyme activity. The end result can lead to a decreased estrogen metabolism, contributing to symptoms and complications due to estrogen dominance.

Notice how I keep stating *can lead to*. My reason for doing so is to once again stress the fact that just because you may have an SNP in your MTHFR gene or COMT gene does not mean you have a problem. Think of your SNPs (and we all have some) as areas where you are more vulnerable. Remember: your genes are not your destiny. The lifestyle you choose to live and the environment you choose to expose your genes to matter most.

The take-home message regarding methylation, SNPs, and Phase 2 estrogen metabolism is that they are directly impacted by our nutritional status, lifestyle behaviors, and environmental exposures. The beauty in all of this, now that we are aware of this information, is we each have the opportunity to modify our diets, lifestyle, and environments to support our estrogen metabolism.

When our Phase 2 enzymes are able to do their job efficiently, our estrogen metabolites are methylated and conjugated, making them less reactive and more water soluble, allowing them to be packaged up within the liver cells and ready for transport into our bile.

Phase 1 and 2 Liver Detoxification

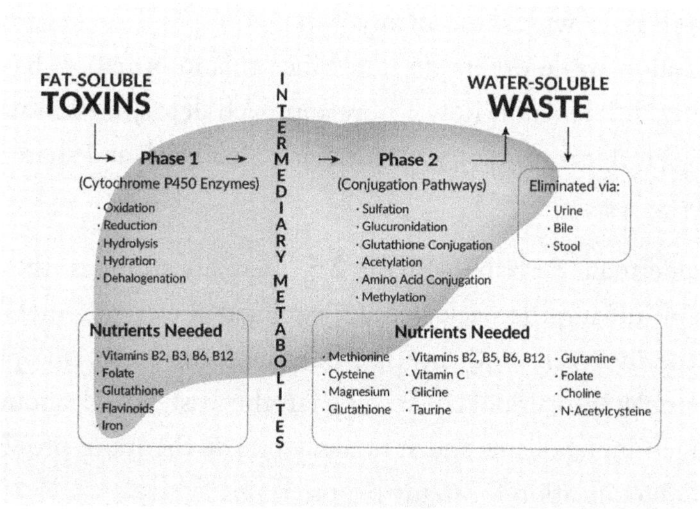

Image #7 – Phase 1 and 2 Liver Detoxification

This brings us to the next phase of estrogen metabolism: Phase 2.5.

Phase 2.5 Detoxification

Once our estrogens have been processed through Phase 1 enzymes (hydroxylation) and packaged-up by Phase 2 enzymes (methylation and conjugation) in our liver, how does our body eliminate them? This brings us to what is now being referred to as *Phase 2.5 Detoxification.*

Many of you may not have heard of Phase 2.5 Detoxification. Honestly, I hadn't either until recently while researching for this book. I was well versed in Phases 1, 2, and 3 detoxification, yet Phase 2.5 was new to me.

I heard the term while listening to an interview with Dr. Kelly Halderman, the academic dean of Kingdom College of Natural Health, regarding estrogen detoxification.[49] I was absolutely amazed by her explanation of what she referred to as *Phase 2.5 Detoxification,* a term she is credited for creating. Her explanation provided me with an answer as to why some of my patients respond so negatively to detoxification while others do not. Since this information has made such a big difference in how I now approach detoxification with my patients, I feel it is necessary to summarize her work and share it with you here.

Dr. Halderman describes Phase 2.5 Detoxification as the actual process of moving the packaged up, conjugated estrogen metabolites out of the liver cells and into the bile. Unfortunately, this phase is often completely overlooked. It is, by far, the least-talked-about phase of estrogen metabolism, and it is likely one of the more problematic areas of detoxification for many people.

Why? Well, Phase 2.5 is intimately connected with and reliant upon two things: the health and function of what are known as our cellular membrane transport proteins, and the health and flow of our bile. As a reminder, our bile is our body's natural built-in hormone and toxin transport system. Healthy bile flow supports healthy hormone elimination. The challenge arises with getting the estrogen metabolites out of the liver cell and into the bile.

Because estrogens were made more water-soluble during Phase 1 and 2 detoxification, and our cell membranes are fat soluble, made up mostly of cholesterol and phospholipids, our estrogens cannot simply diffuse across the cell membrane to get outside the cell and into the bile. Instead, they must be transported across the cell membrane by transport proteins. These transport proteins shuttle more than just estrogens. They also transport toxicants, xenoestrogens, chemicals, medications, drugs, and other hormones out of the cells and into the bile. Therefore, they play a significant role in our overall cellular detoxification.

These transporters are known collectively as *ATP-binding cassettes* (ABCs), and the primary ones impacting estrogen metabolism are *P-glycoproteins*, or *multidrug resistant protein 1* (MRP1) and *multidrug resistant protein 2* (MRP2). The function of these transporters is to act as a shuttle and carry the more water-soluble conjugated estrogens from inside the cell to outside the cell. In the case of MRP1 transporters, the estrogens are deposited outside of the cell into the surrounding interstitial fluid (the fluid bathing the cells) and eventually reenter circulation for elimination via the kidney or bowel. In the case of MRP2 transports, the estrogens are transported out of the liver cell and deposited directly into the bile canaliculi.

Once in the bile, the conjugated estrogens and xenoestrogens flow through the bile ducts and empty into the duodenum of our small intestine through the sphincter of Oddi. Upon entering the small intestine, Phase 3 estrogen detoxification begins. As you will see in the next chapter, it is the health of our intestinal tract and microbiome that ultimately determines the destiny of our conjugated estrogens and xenoestrogens. In the case of a healthy intestine, they are eliminated through bowel movements. Whereas, in the case of an unhealthy intestine, they are more likely to be recycled back into circulation, contributing to estrogen dominance and further toxicity.

Supporting Phase 2.5

Before moving on to Phase 3 estrogen detoxification, let's take a moment and address what it is that impacts our Phase 2.5 Detoxification and why it is such a problematic area of detoxification for many. As mentioned previously, the phases of detoxification, although independent of each other, are interdependent upon each other for overall estrogen metabolism. When it comes to Phase 2.5 Detoxification, the health and function of our cell membranes and transport proteins are paramount. Because our cell membranes are comprised mostly of cholesterol and phospholipids, the amount and types of fats we consume in our daily diet directly impact the health, integrity, and function of the cell membranes.

Higher concentrations of saturated fats, hydrogenated oils, and trans fats result in stiff and rigid cell membranes, making it more difficult to transport items into or out of the cells. Higher concentrations of healthy unsaturated fats, such as olive or avocado oil, or omega-3 fatty acids, result in cell membranes that are much more fluid and flexible. The increased fluidity and flexibility of the cell membranes allow for easier cellular transport and enhance intracellular detoxification. It is much easier to transport estrogens and other toxicants through a flexible cell membrane than a stiff and rigid one.

What Inhibits Our MRP Transporters?

Much like the health of our cell membranes, the ability of our P-glycoprotein transporters to adequately shuttle conjugated estrogens and other toxicants out of our cells and into our bile is critical. The single most potent inhibitor of our P-glycoproteins is chronic inflammation. One of the most common sources of chronic inflammation in our body stems from impaired gut function.

When it comes to impaired gut function, the causes are many (see dysbiosis causes below), yet the end result is often the same: dysbiosis leads to impaired intestinal permeability, or leaky gut. When our gut is leaky, *lipopolysaccharides* (LPS), otherwise known as *endotoxins* (remnants of gram-negative bacteria in our small intestine), leak out of the gut, enter the bloodstream, trigger the release of inflammatory cytokines from the immune cells, and activate the inflammatory cascade. This inflammatory process directly hinders the function of the P-glycoprotein transporters, thus compromising detoxification as a whole. Aside from inflammation, *oxidative stress*, a state of imbalance between the number of free radicals produced within our body and the availability of antioxidants to counteract them, is also an inhibitor of the P-glycoprotein transporters.

Some common causes of dysbiosis and leaky gut:

- Deficiency of stomach acid (hypochlorhydria)
- Deficiency of digestive enzymes
- Deficiency of bile
- Food sensitivities
- Dietary choices
- Decreased intestinal motility
- Existing bowel disease (Crohn's disease, celiac disease, IBD)
- Existing organ dysfunction
- Prior bowel surgery and adhesions
- Medications and antibiotics
- Chronic stress

Free radicals are not necessarily bad. In fact, at low levels, they are important to our overall health.[50] However, many of the dietary and lifestyle choices we make, along with the environmental exposures we encounter, are contributing to very high levels of oxidative stress within our body (see oxidative stress causes below). Such high levels of oxidative stress overwhelm our body by inhibiting our transporters and hindering our natural detoxification processes.

Despite all of this, one fact remains true: Modifying our diet and lifestyle can dramatically reduce our levels of inflammation and oxidative stress. The simplest and easiest way to start this process is by consuming a daily diet rich in organic vegetables and fruits, the recommendation being seven to nine servings daily. This is, by far, the single most effective way to start providing our body with a steady supply of much needed antioxidants.

Some common causes of oxidative stress are:

- Existing disease (obesity, diabetes, cardiovascular disease, and cancer)
- Chronic Infections (H. pylori, EBV, CMV, herpes simplex, Lyme disease)
- A sedentary lifestyle
- Poor diet (high in fat, sugar, and processed foods; low in vegetables, fruits, and fiber)
- Smoking, including vaping and chewing tobacco
- Alcohol consumption
- Medications (prescription and over the counter)
- Poor-quality supplements (fillers, binder)
- Environmental exposure (pesticides, chemicals, toxicants, pollution, metals, radiation)
- Chronic stress
- Disturbed sleep patterns

Silencing Gut Inflammation

In order to maximize the function of our P-glycoproteins, identifying the underlying cause of gut inflammation or oxidative stress is the first step to silencing the inflammatory cascade. This can be challenging—as dysbiosis, leaky gut, and oxidative stress often occur simultaneously—and there are usually multiple causes. This is exactly why looking and going beyond conventional medicine is so important, as there is no pill or procedure to fix these issues.

We need to look through a much broader lens in order to see the bigger picture. We must focus on lifestyle medicine and personalized treatment interventions in order to restore and achieve health. Taking the time to obtain a detailed history and timeline of events is essential. Gathering additional information in the form of questionnaires and surveys is incredibly valuable.

In my office, diet diaries and digestive health surveys are used for every patient. In addition, functional laboratory testing is often necessary to determine the root cause.

Some of the most useful functional tests I use in my office for the evaluation of your gut health are:

- Small intestinal bacterial overgrowth (SIBO) and intestinal methanogen overgrowth (IMO) breath test, to evaluate for dysbiosis

- IBS-Smart test, to evaluate for IBS

- Comprehensive Digestive Stool Analysis (CDSA)with parasitology test, to evaluate gut flora levels, gut function, absorption, inflammation, and the presence of pathogenic microorganisms

- Zonulin, to evaluate the presence of leaky gut

- Food sensitivity IgG testing, to evaluate food intolerances

- Organic Acids Test (OAT), to evaluate overall metabolic health

- Microbiome testing, to determine the richness and diversity of your individual gut microbiome

Some of these tests are now available direct to the consumer, meaning a doctor does not have to order them. Although this provides easier access for testing, interpreting the results correctly is critically important. For best outcomes and treatment options, I recommend you seek out and work with either a naturopathic doctor or a functional or integrative medicine provider.

Caution With Medications

Our discussion on gut health and estrogen metabolism would not be complete without addressing the impact medications can have on your detoxification pathways. Many medications, both prescription and over the counter, are known to inhibit the function of the P-glycoprotein transporters. Let's look at some of the more commonly prescribed classes of prescription medications first.

Antimicrobial agents, macrolide antibiotics (such as clarithromycin and erythromycin), or antifungals (such as ketoconazole or itraconazole) are all potent inhibitors of transport proteins. Many cardiac medications; calcium channel blockers, such as verapamil or diltiazem; beta blockers, such as carvedilol or propranolol; antiarrhythmics, such as amiodarone; and even some statin medications, such as atorvastatin or Lipitor, are potent transport inhibitors.[51]

Many antidepressant medications are also inhibitors. Tricyclic antidepressants, such as Amitriptyline and Doxepin, are also prescribed for nerve pain or sleep disturbance. Selective serotonin reuptake inhibitors (SSRIs), Zoloft, and the selective serotonin and norepinephrine reuptake inhibitors (SSRNI), like Cymbalta, are also potent inhibitors.[52, 53]

Aside from the prescription medications, the ever-increasing use of over-the-counter medications deserves to be addressed as well. PPIs, like Prevacid, Prilosec, and Nexium, are readily available and widely used today. All of them are potent inhibitors of P-glycoprotein transports. I emphasize PPIs here because, in my professional opinion, this is the most dangerous class of medications on the market today. And, to make matters worse, they are readily available over the counter and touted as safe.

While they may be safe when used as intended—up to fourteen days to treat heartburn or acid reflux while seeking to find and address the underlying cause—the problem is they are not being used for just fourteen days as recommended. Even when prescribed by physicians, studies estimate that up to 69 percent of PPI prescriptions are for inappropriate indications.[54] This statistic is in regard to the physician-prescribed PPIs. How many people are self-prescribing now that the medication is available over the counter?

The bottom line is this: This class of medication is not safe for long-term use. Millions of people in the United States and worldwide take PPIs daily and have for years. Prolonged use leads to disastrous long-term negative health consequences, not acknowledged by the conventional medical community.

What are the negative effects? Let's start with a chronic deficiency in stomach acid, leading to impaired protein breakdown, followed by the impaired absorption of essential nutrients such as B12, vitamin C, magnesium, calcium, iron, and zinc. With continued suppression of stomach acid, the onset of dysbiosis and leaky gut, SIBO, fungal overgrowth (candidiasis) is soon to manifest, triggering chronic constipation or diarrhea, onset of food intolerance, impaired gut microbiome, altered systemic pH balance, and systemic inflammation.

Simply put, long-term use of PPIs is not safe. The way in which PPIs are being used today does not heal the gut. Instead, they are used to suppress or cover up symptoms. They are, in truth, distorting our body's pH balance, destroying our microbiome, and compromising the integrity of the entire gut.

Newer research has now linked the long-term use of PPIs with altering gene expression and increasing the risk for kidney disease, Clostridium difficile infection, dementia, increased fracture risk, and overall higher risk of death. As mentioned above, PPIs are not safe for long-term use.

Let's take this one step further and look specifically at the impact PPIs have on estrogen metabolism for a moment. PPIs inhibit every phase of estrogen detoxification. Remember, Phase 1 CYP 450 enzymes are all heme, or iron dependent, and PPIs inhibit the absorption of iron. Our Phase 2 enzymes are B12 and magnesium dependent, and PPIs inhibit the absorption both B12 and magnesium.

The Phase 2.5 transport proteins are directly inhibited by PPIs, and Phase 3 detoxification is dependent on the diversity and health of our microbiome, which is completely distorted by PPIs. The simple truth is that they are not safe medications for any of us to take long term.

What I learned in naturopathic medical school was this: all disease starts in the gut, and all healing starts in the gut.

Identifying and treating the cause for symptoms of indigestion, heartburn, reflux, gas, bloating, belching, or constipation is the answer, not suppressing the symptoms with a medication. In a majority of cases it's the when, how, and what you are eating that causes these symptoms. A PPI is not going to correct that.

For those of you currently taking PPIs, seek support to determine the underlying cause of your symptoms and work with your provider to titrate off the medication. Avoid going *cold turkey* to prevent rebound acid reflux. Your gut, hormones, heart, brain, bones, kidneys, and genes will thank you for it.

As you can see, the healthier our Phase 2.5 detoxification pathway, the more efficient our body is at moving estrogens, xenoestrogen, and toxicants out of our cells and into our bile. Here is where the health of our bile and our bile flow comes into play. This is an area where things can get a bit sticky (no pun intended), and unfortunately, it is a problematic area for many people.

When our bile is thick and sludgy instead of thin and slippery, as it should be, its flow is sluggish. Sluggish or stagnant bile hinders the elimination of estrogens and toxicants. Ensuring healthy bile flow is such a critical step, yet often overlooked, when it comes to successful detoxification (refer to Chapter 3 for the details pertaining to healthy bile and estrogen metabolism). When our bile is healthy and flowing well, it carries estrogens, xenoestrogens, and toxicants out of our liver and empties them into our small intestine for eventual elimination through our bowel. This brings us to location of Phase 3 estrogen metabolism, our intestine, the home of the gut microbiome, which will be addressed in Chapter 5.

Kidney Detoxification

The primary focus of this book is on gut health for hormone balance and detoxification, yet I would be remiss if I did not at least mention the fact that your kidneys also play a role in hormone regulation and detoxification.

Not all our estrogens are excreted via our bile and bowel. Many are eliminated from our body through our kidneys. When the primary transport proteins in our liver are overwhelmed or inhibited, estrogens and toxicants are not transported out of the liver cells into the bile. Instead, they exit our liver cells through a back door, so to speak, entering our bloodstream. They then travel to our kidneys for elimination in our urine.

What is surprising is that the elimination pathways for estrogen and toxicants in the kidneys are very similar to those in our liver. If you recall, the transport proteins in the liver cells act as shuttles to move hormones and toxicants out of the liver cell and into the bile for elimination, while a similar mechanism is at work in our kidneys.

P-glycoprotein transporters within the proximal tubules of our kidneys shuttle estrogens and toxicants from inside the kidney cell out into the urine for elimination. However, the same insults that negatively impact the function of the transport proteins in the liver—inflammation, oxidative stress, and LPS from poor gut health, as well as heavy metals and medications—also inhibit the transport proteins in the kidneys, resulting in decreased elimination of hormones and toxicants.

The underlying message here: maximizing our gut health is key to maintaining healthy functioning liver and kidney transport proteins for hormone balance and detoxification.

Okay. Great job! You did it! You just finished the most complex and complicated section of this book. The volume of information within this chapter may seem overwhelming because much of it may be new to you. You may find going back and reviewing the information again and again helpful. I hope you do. If you find you need further assistance, seek out a naturopathic doctor to assist you.

For those of you more familiar with some of this information—I hope it provides you an even deeper level of understanding. No matter where you may be, I hope I spark your interest and prompt you to take your health to the next level. You may now have a greater appreciation for your liver and all that it does for your body. There is a reason it is known as our body's master detoxification organ.

Chapter 5

Your Gut Microbiome— The Missing Link to Hormone Balance

Patient Case Study: "Amanda"

Amanda, a twenty-five-year-old mother of two small children (ages three and two) was referred to me from her chiropractor after completion of the DUTCH Complete hormone panel in November of 2019 and being informed she was significantly estrogen dominate. She had been self-treating for the prior six months. Our first meeting was in April of 2020.

She shared with me that her menstrual cycles had always been very irregular, anywhere between twenty-one to forty-four days between cycles, ever since starting her menses at age eleven. She had two children and stated both were surprise babies *because her cycles were so irregular. The pregnancies were easy for her, and both babies were full-term home births.*

Following the birth of her second baby, she began noticing changes with her cycle. Despite her cycles being somewhat more regular overall, averaging thirty-three days, she was experiencing significantly worsening PMS symptoms: severe abdominal cramping, anxiety, irritability, headaches, sleep disturbances, and less tolerance for dealing with stress.

Her pain was so intense in November 2018 that she went to the ER. Her abdominal CT scan revealed a mass on her right ovary. The mass was surgically removed and confirmed to be a benign teratoma. Despite the mass removal, Amanda still experienced severe cramping and worsening PMS with her cycle along with more constipation and difficulty losing weight— all symptoms of ongoing estrogen dominance.

This was why her chiropractor ordered the DUTCH panel. Because she was a cycling female, the date of sample collection was important. In order to obtain the most accurate progesterone levels, collecting the sample on days nineteen to twenty-one of the cycle is recommended. Since her cycles were a bit longer, averaging thirty-three days, she collected her sample on the twenty-fourth day of her cycle. Her results showed that her progesterone levels were in the ideal range, yet her estrogen levels, as well as her estrogen metabolites (2-OH and 4-OH), were excessively high for the luteal phase of her cycle.

The DUTCH panel also provided markers indicating she was deficient in B12, B6, and glutathione; thus, she was likely not methylating her estrogens well (an altered Phase 1 and Phase 2 estrogen detoxification). Having constipation was further contributing to her estrogen dominance, as she was not eliminating her estrogens through her bowel movements efficiently (altered Phase 3 estrogen detoxification).

Our initial treatment recommendations included dietary changes to improve her bowel movements. She eliminated gluten, dairy, eggs, and sugar from her diet. I also recommended starting meals with bitters to stimulate her gastric secretion and adding organic cruciferous vegetables and dark leafy greens into her daily diet to support hormone metabolism and gut microbiome.

Organic herbal teas (dandelion root, detox tea, and licorice tea) were recommended to aid with hydration and provide gentle detox support. Supplementation with a probiotic (to support her microbiome), methylated B vitamins (she was low in B12 and B6 on lab testing), chelated magnesium, liposomal glutathione, and a combination product (rich in nutrients and herbs to support her liver in estrogen metabolism) were also added.

I recommended additional lab tests since her last testing had been two years prior. I recommended a full thyroid panel (including antibody levels), a lipid panel, a blood sugar test, a complete metabolic panel, and a complete blood count—all of which were well within the optimal range.

At our six-week follow-up appointment, Amanda reported marked improvement in many areas. She felt eliminating dairy products made the greatest impact on her digestion. She was having daily bowel movements and far fewer headaches, and she stated a 70 percent improvement in PMS and cramping, yet was still concerned about her mood (anxious and weepy) and energy levels. Adrenal support (ashwagandha, or winter cherry) was added to provide her support for both stress and mood.

The plan was to continue tracking her cycle and symptoms; continue her dairy-free, high-fiber diet; and continue her supplement regimen. At the time of her July appointment, Amanda reported she was overall doing and feeling much better. The added adrenal support enhanced her mood and her motivation. Her cycles were becoming more regular, every twenty-eight to thirty days, with minimal PMS and cramping. Our plan was to stay on course and repeat her DUTCH Complete hormone testing in two months.

She completed her testing on day twenty-one of her November cycle, as they had been more regular overall, and we reviewed her results in December. Her labs indicated marked improvement in her level of estrogen dominance, yet now she was slightly low in her levels of overall progesterone. We discussed options for treatment, both natural with diet (seed cycling) and herbs, along with progesterone replacement therapy. Since her symptoms were minor overall, she opted for seed cycling and herbal treatments first.

We also increased her methylated B-vitamin complex to two daily and increased her glutathione (which was still low on her repeat labs) to the full dose of one teaspoon daily. We then scheduled a follow-up appointment in three months.

It is such a pleasure to work with women who are committed to improving their overall health and not looking for a quick fix. Amanda is a great example. She was willing to make the necessary changes to her diet, lifestyle, and self-care practices in order to move from a path of estrogen dominance and potential disease to a path of balance and well-being.

Unlike Phases 1, 2, and 2.5, which mainly occur in our liver, Phase 3 detoxification takes place in our intestinal tract, the home of our gut microbiome. So, what exactly is the *microbiome*? The microbiome is the medical term used to describe all the microorganisms and their genetic material that live within and on our human body. These microorganisms, which are anywhere from ten to fifty times smaller than our own human cells, are composed of archaea, yeasts, viruses, protozoans, and bacteria.

Bacteria, by far, are the most numerous and most studied. For decades, it was estimated that we had ten times more microorganisms living within us and on us then we had actual human cells. This may not actually be the case. Newer research has reported that the once-thought 10:1 ratio of microbes to human cells is far less. Despite that, the biological importance of these microorganisms is what is most important, not necessarily the ratio of cells.[55]

Intense research on the human microbiome began in 2008 with the launching of what is known as the *Human Microbiome Project* (HMP). This project was funded by the National Institute of Health (NIH) and the mission was twofold. First, they wanted to identify and categorize all the microbial communities that live within and on each of us. Second, they wanted to gain a better understanding of how these microbes impact our health and disease.

This fascinating area of scientific research provided insight into the complexities and uniqueness of our microbiome. We learned that each person's microbiome was as unique to that individual as their fingerprint. No two individuals share the same microbiome, not even twins.

From this research, we also gained a greater understanding of the many functions our microbiome performs for us. It supports our body by maintaining the integrity of our intestinal lining (preventing leaky gut), regulating our energy and metabolism, supporting our immunity, balancing our mood, producing vitamins (B12, K) and nutrients (short chain fatty acids), aiding in our digestion and absorption, and playing a critical role in our body's ability to detoxify itself. It is becoming abundantly clear just how vital the gut microbiome is to our overall health.

Now, because the majority of our human microbiome—up to a third—is found in our intestinal tract, this is the site important to Phase 3 detoxification.

How Does the Microbiome Effect Estrogen Metabolism?

What role does the gut microbiome play in regard to estrogen detoxification? Well, to some extent, the health of our gut microbiome actually determines the destiny of our estrogens. When our gut microbiome is healthy and well diversified with balanced levels of microbial stains, the conjugated estrogens and xenoestrogens that were packaged up in our liver (Phases 1 and 2 detox) and sent out through our bile (Phase 2.5 detox) into our intestine are able to pass through our gut microbiome and be eliminated via our bowel moments (Phase 3 detox). Once again, I must stress the importance of having a good bowel movement daily in order to maintain hormone balance.

So, what happens when our gut microbiome is impaired or out of balance (as in the case of SIBO, dysbiosis, leaky gut, or fungal overgrowth)? Ultimately, chronic inflammation ensues, resulting in altered detoxification and hormonal imbalance. Within our gut microbiome, there are several bacterial species that make up what is known as the *estrobolome*. It is the health of our estrobolome which most impacts the levels of our estrogens.

These bacterial species within our estrobolome are capable of producing the enzyme *beta-glucuronidase*, which impacts the metabolism of both estrogens and xenoestrogens. The level of beta-glucuronidase produced within the estrobolome plays a pivotal role in regulating the levels of circulating estrogens and xenoestrogens within our body. We need some beta-glucuronidase enzyme activity because it aids our body in the breakdown of large carbohydrates and assists with the reabsorption of bilirubin.

Maximizing The Microbiome

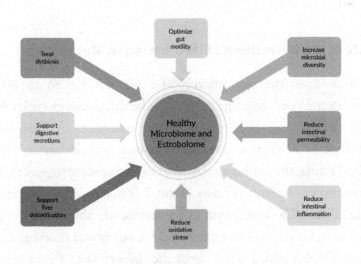

Image #8 – Maximizing The Microbiome

Problems arise when there is an abnormal level of beta-glucuronidase production within the estrobolome. Too much beta-glucuronidase activity predisposes you to recycling too many estrogens and xenoestrogens rather than eliminating them through your bowel. This can eventually lead to the accumulation of both, resulting in a state of estrogen dominance and xenobiotic toxicity, triggering the onset of such conditions as fibrocystic breast, endometriosis, uterine fibroids, and cancers.

How does this happen? During Phase 2 of estrogen detoxification, the liver works hard to methylate and conjugate, or package up, estrogen metabolites into water-soluble molecules so they can be eliminated through the bowel. The beta-glucuronidase enzyme, produced within the estrobolome of our intestine, does the opposite. The enzyme deconjugates, or breaks apart, the conjugated estrogens and xenoestrogens, allowing them to be recycled through enterohepatic circulation.

In essence, high levels of beta-glucuronidase activity simply undo the work your liver had done during Phase 1 and 2 to help rid your body of estrogens and xenoestrogens. Higher levels of circulating estrogen and xenoestrogens are then free to activate estrogen receptors, increase symptoms of hormonal imbalance, and contribute to increased cancer risk.

What Causes High Levels of Beta-Glucuronidase?

The diversity and integrity of our gut microbiome and the composition of our estrobolome are influenced by many factors. Our genetics do play a role, yet only a small one. Interestingly, genetic factors account for only about 10 percent of the variation in our gut microbiota.[56] What about the remaining 90 percent? This is where epigenetics come into the picture.

If you recall, epigenetics is the field of study addressing how our environment interacts with our genes. Both our individual environment and our global environmental factors impact not only our microbiome, but also our genes and how they are expressed.

Up until the mid-1990s, science really knew very little about the microbiome. It's only been over the last twenty years that this field of study has been growing. Research and science clearly show that changes to our microbiome and estrobolome can impact beta-glucuronidase enzyme levels and activity.

We directly and negatively impact the diversity and integrity of our gut microbiome through the following:

- Dietary and lifestyle behaviors
- Use of medication (both prescription and over the counter)
- Chronic stress
- Altered sleep cycles
- Physical inactivity
- Systemic inflammation
- Toxin exposures

The good news is that all of the above-mentioned factors are modifiable. Through lifestyle and dietary interventions, each of us has the opportunity to improve our gut microbiome, restore our hormone balance, and prevent many of the chronic diseases seen in our world today. When it comes to our gut microbiome, what is truly surprising is just how receptive and responsive it is to dietary changes. We once thought it would take weeks or even months to change our microbiome, yet we now know that is simply not the case. Making a big dietary shift (for example, moving to a plant-based diet from an animal-based diet) can change the levels of our gut bacteria and the kinds of genes they express in as little as three to four days.

How Do I Know If My Gut Microbiome Is Impaired?

There are numerous studies showing the diversity of our gut microbiome is associated with both gut health and overall health, while a lack of diversity in our microbiome tends toward ill health and disease.

How do you know if your microbiome is healthy or not? Check in with yourself and see if you are experiencing some of the following symptoms or conditions. If so, the health of your gut microbiome may be a contributing factor.

Gastrointestinal symptoms:

- Abdominal pain
- Bloating and gas
- Constipation
- Diarrhea
- Food poisoning
- Gastritis
- Gastroenteritis
- Gastroesophageal reflux (GERD)
- Small intestinal bacterial overgrowth (SIBO)
- Ulcers
- Vomiting

Associated autoimmune conditions:

- Crohn's Disease
- Ulcerative Colitis
- Gastric Cancer
- Ankylosing Spondylitis
- Reactive and Rheumatoid Arthritis
- Thyroiditis (Hashimoto's, Graves')

Associated allergic conditions:

- Asthma
- Eczema

Associated metabolic diseases:

- Obesity
- Diabetes
- Atherosclerosis
- Cancer

Diversity and Balance Really Do Matter

Have you ever wondered why some people can eat larger amounts of food and stay thin while others eat tiny portions and still gain weight? Well, believe it or not, the health of their microbiome may be a contributing factor. The bacteria in our gut not only play an important role in our digestion and absorption, but research also shows that our microbiome plays a major role in whether we become overweight and obese.

The findings from the Human Microbiome Project revealed that our gut microbiome comprises 500-1000 different bacterial species, which have been classified into twelve different phyla (or families) of bacteria.[57] Of the twelve, two phyla, the *Firmicutes* and *Bacteroidetes*, make up nearly 90 percent of our entire gut microbiome.[58] The ratio between these two phyla in our gut can impact both our body weight and our levels of inflammation.

When the ratio of Firmicutes to Bacteroidetes is out of balance, we are far more likely to gain weight. Why? Firmicutes play a role in regulating how much fat we absorb from our diet, and they thrive on sugar. Our current Western diet, which is rich in both fat and sugar, not only feeds the Firmicutes well, but also promotes an imbalanced ratio of Firmicutes to Bacteroidetes. And a higher ratio further enhances the absorption of our dietary fats and sugars, resulting in weight gain and obesity.

What is a potential solution? You guessed it: modifying our diet and lifestyle to support our microbiome balance.

Five Simple Ways to Restore Your Firmicutes/Bacteroidetes Ratio

There are five simple ways to restore your Firmicute/Bacteroidetes ratio:

1. Eliminate sugar, alcohol, and processed foods.

2. Increase your daily consumption of high-fiber foods—gut flora feed on fiber.

3. Add fermented foods into your daily diet—they are rich in natural probiotics.

4. Incorporate more beans into your daily diet.

   a. Beans are among the very best foods to raise your level of Bacteroidetes.

   b. Train your bacteria to digest beans well by adding in small amounts (about a tablespoon) to your diet every two to three days, and gradually increasing the amount.

5. Establish a sleep schedule and an eating schedule.

   a. Similar to our sleep/wake cycle, our gut microbiome changes rhythm throughout the day. Our microbiome, like most of us, is most efficient and productive during the daylight hours. Erratic mealtimes, late-night shift work, and jet lag disrupt our microbial rhythm and impair our healthy gut bacteria much the same as antibiotics do.

b. Incorporate intermittent fasting as part of your lifestyle to support your microbiome, reduce inflammation, and balance your circadian rhythm. (See intermittent fasting section below.)

As mentioned previously, weight gain and obesity are common outcomes resulting from a lack of microbial diversity and balance. Unfortunately, with weight gain and obesity comes higher levels of chronic inflammation.

Our adipocytes, or fat cells, release what are known as *cytokines*, or inflammatory triggers. These cytokines activate our immune cells and disrupt our insulin function, contributing to what is known as *insulin resistance*. Insulin resistance leads to altered glucose metabolism, which further perpetuates weight gain and inflammation. This vicious cycle continues over and over again. The more adipose tissue we have, the more chronically inflamed we are likely to be.

Inflammation is often touted as the underlying trigger for all chronic diseases seen today, yet how does it negatively impact your estrogen metabolism?

Here are some ways estrogen metabolism is hindered by chronic inflammation:

1. In the lymphatics, inflammation diminishes flow, resulting in lymphatic stagnation and fluid retention.

2. In the gallbladder, inflammation increases bile sludge and gallstone formation and reduces bile flow.

3. In the liver, inflammation reduces enzyme activity in both Phase 1 and Phase 2 detoxification and suppresses the function

of our transport proteins in Phase 2.5, directly inhibiting the metabolism of estrogen and xenoestrogens.

4. In the intestine, inflammation leads to malabsorption, food intolerances, leaky gut, fungal overgrowth, dysbiosis, IBS, and SIBO, further perpetuating inflammation.

5. In the microbiome, inflammation alters gut flora diversity and balance, contributing to higher beta-glucuronidase activity and estrogen/xenoestrogen recycling.

Can the Microbiome and Beta-Glucuronidase Levels Be Tested?

Thanks to advances in technology such as next-generation sequencing and the rise of *metagenomics* (the study of microbial communities), it is now possible for you to have your microbiome tested. As you may have guessed, stool samples are required for such testing. The cost of gut microbiome testing significantly varies depending upon the extent of the testing provided. The turnaround time for most lab results is generally two to four weeks.

Let me say: test results can be complex and complicated. Therefore, I highly recommend you work with a qualified provider (a naturopathic doctor, functional medicine, or integrative practitioner) in order to achieve the best outcome. There are now several laboratory companies offering microbiome testing and some sell directly to the health consumer. A few microbiome testing companies include:

- Viome Gut Intelligence Test
- Biome Gut Test
- Thryve Gut Health Test
- GI MAP Test by Diagnostics Solutions Laboratory
- GI Effects Test by Genova Diagnostics
- GI 360 Microbiome Profile by Doctor's Data

Can I Restore My Microbiome to Maximize Estrogen Metabolism?

In order to restore and maintain our microbiome, we need to know why and how it became impaired in the first place. For some of us, it may date back to the time of our birth. If you were fortunate enough to be born via vaginal delivery and were breast fed as a newborn, your microbiome was off to a great start. Being inoculated with microbes during the birthing process and while breast feeding has shown to be a key foundational factor for our overall microbiome health.

Unfortunately, growing up and living in today's world, our gut microbiome endures repeated daily insults through our dietary, lifestyle, and environment exposures. I've listed my top ten suggestions for you to begin the process of restoring and maintaining a healthy microbiome below:

1. Move away from Western-style diets, also known as the Standard American Diet (SAD).

2. Incorporate intermittent fasting into your daily lifestyle.

3. Strive to eat clean and organic food as much as possible and go green by using products safe for your environment.

4. Critically evaluate the need and use of medications.

5. Identify and address your daily stressors.

6. Make your sleep routine a priority.

7. Move your body—movement is medicine.

8. Identify your food intolerances and sensitivities.

9. Address and correct your digestive impairments.

10. Supplement key nutrients when necessary.

As you can see from the list above, the health of our gut microbiome can be dramatically impacted by our daily choices. Choosing wisely is paramount to a healthy gut, and a healthy gut is paramount to healthy hormones.

When it comes specifically to lowering beta-glucuronidase activity in our gut, the foods we choose to eat can make a difference. Many foods are rich in a substance known as *glucaric acid*. When combined with calcium, it becomes calcium-D-glucarate.

Calcium-D-glucarate is important because it reduces beta-glucuronidase activity, thereby reducing the recycling and enhancing the elimination of estrogens and xenoestrogens through our bowel. Calcium-D glucarate is commonly sold as an over-the-counter nutritional supplement for treatment and prevention of hormone imbalance, but it's still best to use food first whenever possible.

While taking calcium-D-glucarate as a supplement may help lower beta-glucuronidase activity, it does not effectively change the microbiome. Therefore, it does not actually reduce the production of beta-glucuronidase. Instead, it works by decreasing the activity of the beta-glucuronidase enzyme. Real food, on the other hand, rich in fiber and other nutrients, has the ability to modify the microbiome and the estrobolome, thereby reducing the overall production of the beta glucuronidase enzyme. Just another example of how our food can be powerful medicine. The more diverse our food intake—particularly plants—on a daily basis, the more diverse and balanced our gut microbiome is likely to be.

Food sources that can enhance calcium-D-glucarate include:[59]

- Legumes: cooked or sprouted mung beans and adzuki bean sprouts

- Fruits: oranges, grapefruits, lemons, sweet cherries, grapes, apples, peaches, plums, apricots

- Vegetables: spinach, carrots, alfalfa sprouts, cabbage, Brussels sprouts, cauliflower, broccoli, corn, cucumber, lettuce, celery, green pepper, tomato, and potatoes

As you can see, restoring and maintaining a healthy, balanced, and well-diversified microbiome takes effort. It requires conscious thought, consistent behavior, and continuous self-surveillance. A good place to start is by tuning in and asking yourself: *How am I doing today? How am I feeling today?*

Personal responsibility is the tipping point in the process of removing chronic insults and replacing them with nourishing nutrients and behaviors. I refer to this process as *incorporating daily detoxification practices*. In Chapter 11, I'll discuss how you can move forward with incorporating detoxification practices into your daily routines.

Is Intermittent Fasting a Sure Way to Support Gut Health and Hormone Balance?

I want to address the benefits intermittent fasting can offer to your overall health; specifically, how it can benefit hormone balance. The term *intermittent fasting* is more of an umbrella term, as it encompasses a few different types of fasting.

There are three different types of intermittent fasting: alternate-day fasting, periodic fasting, and time-restricted feeding.

Although I discuss all three types of intermittent fasting with my patients, the type I routinely recommend is time-restricted feeding. Why is this my go-to? For two reasons.

First, time-restricted feeding is the easiest for most people to follow and tolerate, since they are able to choose their eating window. Second, time-restricted feeding, unlike the other types, has a greater impact on your circadian rhythm, also known as our internal clock, which regulates our sleep/wake cycle and hormones.

For those of you interested in learning more about intermittent fasting, I highly recommend a book By Dr. Jason Fong, *The Complete Guide to Fasting*, which provides much greater detail on the different types of fasting and associated health benefits.

What Exactly Is Time-Restricted Feeding?

Think of it this way: we all have twenty-four hours in a given day, and most of us have the ability to choose when we eat. Time-restricted feeding simply means carving out a daily designated eight-to-twelve-hour eating window. We all know that *what* we eat is obviously important to our health, yet *when* we choose to eat can also have significant impacts on our health as well.

With time-restricted feeding, the goal is to create an eight-to-twelve-hour eating window, followed by a twelve-to-sixteen-hour fasting window that works best for you and your lifestyle. For example, some may choose a 10:00 a.m.–6:00 p.m. feeding window, in which they skip breakfast (drinking plain black coffee, tea, or water is acceptable while fasting) and then eat lunch and dinner. This eating window seems to work well for many people, as it allows them to still have dinner with their family.

For those of you who really enjoy breakfast, maybe a 6:00 a.m.–2:00 p.m. or 8:00 a.m.–4:00 p.m. feeding window may work best. The timing of your specific eating window is not necessarily what's most important (except for late night eating, which I discuss in the microbiome chapter). What's most important here is finding the right eating window that works for you, your body, and your lifestyle, and sticking to it.

Consistency is the key to success!

Think of your eating window more as a lifestyle behavior, much like brushing your teeth. Incorporating an eating window in your daily routine allows it to become a habit over time. To maximize the benefits of your efforts, choose your eating window such that you allow for as close as possible to a three-hour period of fasting before going to bed. Going to bed on a full stomach is not conducive to a good night of restorative sleep; it also disrupts hormone levels.

Time-restricted feeding is beneficial to your overall health and hormone balance for many reasons, but I want to stress five primary benefits.

Time-restricted feeding:

1. Positively impacts your body's *sirtuin proteins*. Sirtuin proteins are a family of seven proteins, SIRT 1 to SIRT 7, that play a key role in regulating your body's overall homeostasis, or cellular balance. These proteins are responsible for repairing your DNA and ultimately protecting you against the development of cancer. It is not surprising that the sirtuin proteins, in particular SIRT 6, have often been referred to as *your body's natural longevity genes*. The challenge is that the only way to activate and tap into the benefits of sirtuin proteins is by putting your body into a fasting state.

2. Positively impacts your body's natural circadian rhythm by enhancing your body's metabolism and energy expenditure.

3. Stabilizes your blood sugar and insulin levels, thus significantly lowering your risk of obesity, diabetes, and one of the most rapidly occurring conditions, nonalcohol fatty liver disease. Research shows that the timing of your calorie consumption does, indeed, matter. Insulin sensitivity, meaning how

efficiently it works to regulate your blood sugar, decreases throughout the day.[60] Therefore, eating earlier, during the day, rather than later, during the evening hours, may be most beneficial.

4. Maximizes your microbiome diversity and function, dramatically reducing gut permeability (or leaky gut), postprandial endotoxemia [or the intestinal absorption of gut lipopolysaccharides (LPS) after eating], and systemic inflammation.

5. Allows your gut to cleanse itself by activating what is known as the *migrating motor complex* (MMC) in the upper gastrointestinal tract. The MMC is a cyclic, recurring motility pattern, occurring about every ninety minutes in your stomach and small intestine while in a fasting state. Think of the MMC as your intestinal housekeeper cyclically sweeping undigested matter and other contents into the large intestine, helping to maintain a healthy balance of intestinal flora.

What does all this have to do with hormone balance? Your body's ability to metabolize estrogens and eliminate them, along with other toxins, is highly dependent upon the health and function of your gut, your liver, and your microbiome. Incorporating time-restricted feeding into your daily lifestyle positively impacts all three areas and is one sure way toward restoring and maintaining your hormone balance.

Another benefit: it doesn't cost a thing.

Part Two

What You Need to Do

Chapter 6

The Removal and Replacement Process

Removal Process

The removal process is likely to be the most challenging step for you. This is where you'll need to *let go and get rid of* the things you discover are not serving you on your quest for hormone balance and better health. Often this is easier said than done, as this requires changes in many areas of your life. Everything from your diet and routines to your habits and hobbies.

Please remember that this is a process—a lifestyle change, and not a quick fix—and it's best done in stages, not all at once. Success breeds success, and you build upon your success one accomplishment at a time.

II liken it to the principle of *Feng Shui*. In terms of Feng Shui, this would be the equivalent of *clearing your clutter*. Doing so invites and allows the flow of energy and vitality. Cleaning up your diet, your lifestyle, and your personal environment affords your body the opportunity to repair, regenerate, restore, and renew.

Why? You are lowering your body's overall toxic load. I can honestly say that if you are alive today you are probably toxic. There is no way to completely avoid toxins. They are in the food you eat, the water you drink, the air you breathe, the environments where you live, your habits, the hobbies you engage in, and your profession. Toxins are simply everywhere.

Despite all of this, do not lose hope! There are choices you can make each and every day to reduce your toxic exposure. That is your first goal: reducing your daily exposure. There are choices you can make daily to support your body in eliminating the toxins already present within. Your second goal is to incorporate daily detoxification practices. The combination of reducing exposure and enhancing detoxification, in particular maximizing you gut health, is the primary way to restore your hormones and bring your health back into balance.

Below I have listed the six key areas, and the five components of each area, that I share with all my patients in clinical practice. It may seem like a lot, but as a naturopathic doctor, I treat you—your whole person—not just your symptoms. The less exposure you have to any of the following, the healthier your gut will be and the happier your hormones will be. We all have areas we can improve upon. What areas most apply to you?

Food: Medicine or Poison?

Food is always a great place to start from the naturopathic perspective, as we are true believers in this idea often attributed to Hippocrates: "Let thy food be thy medicine and thy medicine be thy food." The problem is that most food today is not at all what it used to be. In fact, I would go as far and say that some of what we call food isn't even food at all—for example, soda pop.

Most of what we eat today has been processed, manipulated, modified, engineered, exposed to pesticides, or fortified in ways that has turned the food into potential poisons for your body.

Let's take a look at how and why food choices contribute to impaired gut health, ultimately contributing to altered detoxification and hormone imbalance.

1. **Processed food and artificial sweeteners**: These lack nutrients and lead to nutritional deficiencies, weight gain, and impaired gut microbiome balance, diversity, and integrity. All of this leads to poor detoxification and hormonal imbalance.

2. **High in sugar or fructose**: These lack nutrients and are high in calories, contributing to weight gain. They also significantly prolong gut transit time, increase hydrogen gas production, and alter gut function and bowel bacteria composition. Glucose or fructose induces changes in gut microbiome, gut permeability, and inflammation and promotes fatty liver accumulation.

3. **Nonorganic (conventional) fruits and vegetables**: Most are treated with pesticides (mostly organophosphates), found to perturb the gut microbiome community structure.

4. **Farm-raised animals and animal products**: Consumption of animal products, particularly dairy products derived from pregnant cows, has been associated with breast, ovarian, and uterine cancers. High animal-protein diets result in lower Bifidobacterium levels and less short chain fatty acids (SCFAs) production, increasing the risk of inflammatory bowel disease (IBD). High-protein diets are associated with higher levels of beta-glucuronidase levels, contributing to altered estrogen metabolism.

5. **Genetically Modified Foods**: 85 to 95 percent of genetically modified (GM) crops worldwide are treated with glyphosate, which is now known to directly distort the diversity of function of the gut microbiome.

Lifestyle: The Way You Live Your Life Matters

The science is crystal clear: your lifestyle matters.

How important is it? As mentioned in Chapter 1, the WHO reported in 2018 that chronic disease (diabetes, obesity, cardiovascular disease, and cancer) now surpasses infectious disease as the number one cause of death worldwide. Additionally, the CDC reports that the top four factors contributing to this shift are poor nutrition, lack of physical activity, smoking, and alcohol. All of these are modifiable factors.

Some 80 percent of all healthcare costs are related to chronic diseases, and 80 percent of all chronic disease is related to lifestyle choices. This is huge! When it comes to your health, the choices you make each day can either lead you down the path toward health and well-being or down the path toward illness and disease.

Here are some lifestyle factors to consider:

1. **Sedentary Lifestyle**: This has been reported by the World Health Organization to be one of the top three risk factors for all chronic disease.[61] It contributes to overall reduced gastrointestinal function, slower bowel transit time impacting the diversity and function of microbiome, higher risk for gallstones, and nonalcohol fatty liver disease, directly inhibiting detoxification and altered hormone metabolism.

2. **Chronic Stress**: Significantly disrupts microbiome diversity (lowering levels of Lactobacillus), reduces SCFA production, and increases colonic inflammation.

3. **Disturbed Sleep**: Altered circadian rhythm (sleep-wake cycle), sleep deprivation, and late shift work have been shown to negatively change the structure and diversity of the gut microbiome.

4. **Electromagnetic Fields (EMFs)**: In today's modern world, we are surrounded by EMFs: power lines, smart meters, computer devices, televisions, radios, and telephones. These have destructive effects on sex hormones, gonadal function, fetal development, and pregnancy. Some of us are more susceptible to the effects of EMFs based on our body weight, body-mass index, bone density, and hydration and electrolytes status, which can alter the conductivity of and biological reactivity to EMFs. Cell phone level RF-EMF disrupts human skin microbiota, and this finding can lay the ground for more research on the effect of RF-EMF on human health through the human-microbiota relationship.

5. **Toxic Relationships and People**: Both will hinder your mental, emotional, and physical well-being contributing to stress. Chronic stress has shown to negatively impact microbiome diversity and function.

Environment: Your Genes' Environment Impacts Their Expression

There is no way around it—you are living in a toxic world, and it's negatively affecting your gut, hormones, and overall health. Chemicals known as *endocrine disrupting compounds* surround you in your daily life, often without your even knowing it.

They can be found in:

- Food you eat
- Air you breathe
- Water you drink
- Home you live in
- Buildings you work in
- Hobbies you engage in

These chemicals disrupt the normal function and activity of your adrenal hormones, thyroid hormones, and sex hormones (estrogen, progesterone, and testosterone). They can also deplete your body of essential vitamins, minerals, antioxidants, and neurotransmitters, contributing to a host of added health problems.

Most of us were led to believe that our genetics determine our destiny. What science—the field of epigenetics in particular—tells us is that the environment we put our genes in is what really matters.

Let's take a closer look:

1. **Dirty (unfiltered) air**: The average person breathes in approximately 11,000 liters of air per day. That's a lot of potential for toxin exposure, including smog, particulate matter, heavy metals, ozone, volatile organic compounds (VOCs), and mold. Additionally, the Environmental Protection Agency (EPA) reports that air quality inside homes and buildings may be more seriously polluted than the air outside, even in cities. Combine this with the fact that most people spend 90 percent of their time indoors.[62]

2. **Dirty (unfiltered) water**: Heavy metals, pesticides, VOCs, and pharmaceutical drugs have all been detected in the water supply. Each adds to our body's burden and compromises our detoxification pathways.

3. **Plastics**: Phthalates and bisphenol A plastics are all around us—in food packaging, storage containers, plastic water bottles—and are all classified as hormone-disrupting chemicals associated with increased risk for breast, ovarian, and prostate cancers.

4. **Toxic personal care products**: Toxic ingredients such as paraben, fragrances, phthalates, formaldehyde, mercury,

lead, and cadmium are shown to be endocrine disruptors and carcinogenic, or cancer producing.

5. **Toxic household cleaners**: The average household contains approximately sixty-two toxic chemicals, many linked to asthma, cancer, reproductive disorders, hormone disruption, and neurotoxicity.[63] Chronic exposure adds to our body's toxic burden, compromising our natural detoxification pathways.

Habits: Your Routine Is Important

Your habits are behaviors or activities you do without really thinking twice about it. Chewing your nails when feeling nervous, for example. Yet some habits are detrimental to your health, and if continued long term, can lead to addiction. For example, what started out as an occasional glass of wine with a friend or loved one can easily become a necessity at the end of the day, just to settle down from the stress of life. Before you know it, one glass is no longer enough: it takes two or more glasses to do the trick.

I use this exact example because I see it so often in clinical practice. Ladies tend to love their wine (or other alcohol), but what they don't know is the detrimental impact chronic alcohol has on their gut health, hormone health, and overall health for that matter. Remember, when it comes to your health, the choices you make each day can either lead you down the path toward health and well-being or down the path toward illness and disease.

1. **Tobacco**: The WHO has reported tobacco as one of the top-three risk factors for all chronic disease. Smoking contributes to modifications of the oral, lung, and gut microbiome, leading to various diseases, such as periodontitis, asthma, chronic obstructive pulmonary disease, Crohn's disease, ulcerative colitis, and cancers. The use of **e-cigarettes** and **vaping** are

not safer alternatives. The chronic repetitive exposure to e-cigarette aerosols disrupts the gut epithelial barrier, increases the susceptibility of the gut lining to bacterial infections, and triggers gut inflammation.[64]

2. **Alcohol**: Alcohol is another of the top-three risk factors, according to the WHO. Alcohol directly disrupts estrogen and xenoestrogen detoxification pathways in our liver and contributes to the onset of cancer. It also directly impairs the gut microbiome and contributes to the development of gut inflammation and SIBO.

3. **Frequent cannabis use**: Chronic cannabis use can have suppressive effects on the adrenal glands, thyroid gland, and reproductive systems for both men and women, and can potentially affect energy, behavior, and reproductive health.[65] Chronic cannabis use can suppress ovulation, leading to lower progesterone levels contributing to estrogen dominance.

4. **Night-time snacking**: Late-night eating results in a significant alternation in the compositions and functions of our gut microbiota, which further contributes to the development of metabolic disorders.

5. **Excess caffeine**: This has been shown to disrupt the circadian clock (sleep-wake cycle), delaying onset of sleep. Caffeine, found in coffee, tea, and other foods, can induce a response in our neuroendocrine stress pathways, which are known to interact with the microbiota.

Medications: More Harm Than Good?

The use of medications is at an all-time high. Over the past twenty years, the total number of prescriptions filled by all Americans (for adults *and* children) have increased by 85 percent, while the population has only increased by 21 percent.[66] Medications that were once only available by prescription are now easily accessible over the counter. All medications, prescription and OTC, must be taken seriously.

Medications are most often treating symptoms and not addressing the underlying cause. Although common side effects of medications may be addressed, the silent side effects are almost never addressed.

What are silent side effects of medications? I am referring to what I describe as *medication-induced nutritional deficiencies.* Medications deplete vital nutrients over time.

A few common examples are:

- **Metformin**: Used for blood sugar regulation; it depletes vitamin B12.

- **Statins**: Used for lowering cholesterol (e.g., Crestor, Lipitor); they deplete CoQ10, vitamin D, and beta-carotene.

- **Antidepressants**: SSRIs deplete calcium and vitamin D.

Unfortunately, medications are often concurrently taken with other medications, further compounding nutrient deficiencies. One thing to keep in mind here is that all medications need to be metabolized and excreted from your body, and this puts significant strain on your detoxification organs—specifically your liver, microbiome, and kidneys. Also keep in mind that OTC medications can be equally as dangerous as prescription medications.

Some other examples are:

1. **Proton Pump Inhibitors (PPIs)**: Chronic treatment with PPIs strongly impacts small intestine microbiota due to loss of the gastric acid defensive barrier, which causes small intestinal bacterial overgrowth (SIBO). PPIs enhance the expression of bacteria with beta-glucuronidase activity, encouraging the

enterohepatic recycling of estrogens and xenoestrogens. PPIs reduce gastric acid secretion, resulting in profound changes in the colonic microbiota with a reduction in overall microbial diversity. PPIs deplete our body of magnesium, calcium, iron, zinc, vitamin C, and B12.

2. **Non-Steroidal Anti-Inflammatory Drugs (NSAIDs)**: With NSAIDs, impact on bacterial composition varies depending on the specific medication used. NSAIDs used in combination with PPIs is not a good idea, as PPIs have been reported to exacerbate the mucosal damage caused by NSAIDs in the distal portion of the small bowel. Also, NSAIDs deplete the body of iron and vitamin C.

3. **Antibiotics**: There is ample evidence that antibiotic use reduces gut microbial diversity, balance, and abundance.[67]

4. **Synthetic Estrogens (ethinyl estradiol)**: Your liver cytochrome P-450 enzymes (needed for Phase 1 estrogen metabolism), the chief site of oxidative transformation of ethinyl estradiol, can become irreversibly inactivated by the intermediate compounds of ethinyl estradiol metabolism. Estrogens deplete the body of B vitamins (6, 12, and folate), vitamins C and E, calcium, and magnesium.

5. **Birth Control Pills (BCPs)**: Estrogens and oral contraceptives are both associated with several liver-related complications, including intrahepatic cholestasis, sinusoidal dilatation, peliosis hepatitis, hepatic adenomas, hepatocellular carcinoma, hepatic venous thrombosis, and an increased risk of gallstones.[68] BCPs deplete the body of B vitamins (6, 12, folate), vitamin C and E, calcium, and magnesium.

Hobbies: Your Hobbies May Expose You to Unknown Toxins

Many of you have hobbies you enjoy doing, and I encourage you to do so. Having a hobby can provide a lot of positives: relaxation, developing new skills, staying active and physically fit, and maybe some additional income. Regardless of the reasons you choose to pursue your hobbies, I ask you to consider taking some time to evaluate potential exposures you may be coming into contact with. Once you're aware of what you're dealing with, you can take the necessary steps to eliminate, or at least reduce, your risk of exposure. Let's take a look at a few examples of potential toxins associated with some common hobbies.

1. **Painting (oil or spray)**: The paint you're using may contain heavy metals (lead, cadmium, nickel) and VOCs (like solvents and formaldehyde), which could be inhaled or swallowed, posing health risks.

2. **Stained glass**: Dust from *lead cames* used in stained glass can be inhaled and swallowed, posing a health risk.

3. **Jewelry making**: You can be exposed to heavy metals (cadmium and lead), solvents, and sealants, which pose health risks.

4. **Refinishing furniture**: Many woods are pretreated with pesticides and preservatives. Also, VOCs (such as paint thinner, turpentine, toluene, xylene, and alcohols) pose health risks.

5. **Golf**: Synthetic fertilizers, herbicides, insecticides, fungicides, and other chemicals used on the greens may pose health risks.

The changes you make in these six key areas over time can significantly lower your body's toxic exposure and lessen your body's overall toxic burden. Even *small* changes in a *few* areas can synergistically make a big difference. Remember: decreasing your body's exposure and lowering your body's toxic burden are the goals in the removal process. Doing so allows your body's natural detoxification pathway to function more efficiently. While it can be difficult to remove substances from your life (even when you know those things are not good for you), the process of removal is easier and much more successful when you have something else to replace those items with.

This brings you to the next step in the process: replacing and replenishing.

The Replacing and Replenishing Process

Below, I've listed simple, healthful, easy-to-incorporate, and meaningful ways to make changing these areas of your lifestyle a little easier:

Food Is Medicine

Natural sweeteners will always be a better choice when used in moderation:

- **Honey**: Perhaps the oldest sweetener known to humankind, it has antimicrobial properties and contains nondigestible fiber. Honey serves as prebiotic and selectively modulates the gut microbial balance by inducing probiotic lactobacilli and Bifidobacteria.

- **Blackstrap molasses**: Aside from being rich in iron, calcium, magnesium, manganese, potassium, selenium, and vitamin B6, it also may enhance your body's natural anti-inflammatory response by modulating the microbiome.

- **Maple syrup**: Aside from containing potassium, calcium, magnesium, and vitamins B2 and B3, it is rich in nondigestible fibers (inulin, dextran, arabinogalactan, and rhamnogalacturonan), all known to benefit the modulation of the gut microbiome.

- **Coconut palm sugar**: This has a low glycemic index due to its inulin (a soluble fiber) content. Inulin is a prebiotic known to benefit the modulation of the gut microbiome.

- **Stevia**: Highly popular due to being noncaloric and considered safe up to 4 mg/kg daily, it may not offer microbiome benefits.

Clean food is essential to life. Here's where you can find it:

- **Go organic.** The controversy between conventional versus organically grown food is not whether or not one form is more nutritious than the other. The true controversy concerns the levels of known toxins used in the growing and harvesting of our conventional food supply. Mounting evidence supports the detrimental effects the toxins in our food supply (whether from herbicides, pesticides, preservatives, chemicals, additives, or hormones) have on our microbiome, hormone balance, and overall health.

  - One solution to consider is to grow your own food, or at least some of your own food, using only natural fertilizers and sprays as necessary. Talk about wholesome and fresh—you can't get much better than home grown.

  - Another option is to shop at the farmers' markets or food co-ops in your area. It is a win-win: good for them and good for you.

- **Fill up on fiber and phytonutrients.** The single best way to maximize your microbiome function is to feed it fiber, as this is the primary fuel for your gut flora. You want to strive to eat seven to nine servings of organic vegetables and fruits a day.

- **Diversity matters**. In 2018, the results of the American Gut Project (a global citizen science effort) were published. They showed that participants eating more than thirty different plant types per week had more diverse gut microbiomes than those who ate ten or fewer types of plants per week.[69] The bottom line is that the more diverse the intake of plants in our daily diet, the greater the diversity of our microbiome.

- **Introduce fermented foods into your daily diet**. Fermented foods and beverages help provide a spectrum of probiotics to foster a vigorous microbiome and cause significant positive improvements in balancing intestinal permeability and barrier function, thus lessening the risk for leaky gut.

  - The beauty is that many types of food groups—dairy, vegetables, fruits, legumes, grains, starchy roots, as well as meat and fish—can be fermented, so there is a little something for everyone's taste.

  - A little goes a long way. I recommend starting with one small serving—one tablespoon of sauerkraut or kimchi per day.

- **Incorporate intermittent fasting**. Establish a routine of eating outside a twelve-to-sixteen-hour window of fasting (water and herbal teas are okay) each day.

Lifestyle

Movement is medicine. There is no doubt about it—exercise and physical activity positively impact every single body system, including your microbiome.

- I will borrow the slogan once used by the athletic apparel company, Nike, and say—*Just Do It*. Find what it is you like to do, and just do it!

- Remember, it is the consistency of your physical activity that makes the greatest impact, not necessarily the type of the physical activity you choose.

Decompress from stress. Stress is a part of life and managing it is the key. Learn to check in with yourself intermittently throughout the day. Stress has a way of sneaking up on us. Seek to determine what triggers your stress and how it affects your body. What is your body trying to tell you?

- Much like exercise, find what works best to negate your stress and build it into your day. The examples listed below cost very little or nothing at all. They can all be incorporated easily into a daily routine.

  - Examples: stretching, deep breathing, mindfulness, meditating, yoga, aromatherapy (essential oils), music, being in nature, journaling, laughing, dancing, spending time with others or pets, setting boundaries, taking a bath, learning to say "no," and talking about how you're feeling.

- Supplementation may be helpful when dealing with chronic stress, as stress can induce nutritional deficiencies, which, in turn, make it more difficult to handle stressors.

My top three nutrients for supporting the body with stress include:

- **Omega-3 fatty acids** – shown to reduce both inflammation and anxiety in young, healthy individuals when administered prior to stressful events.

- **Magnesium** – often referred to as our *anti-stress mineral,* but it is lost through our urine at an accelerated rate during periods of prolonged stress.

- **B vitamins** – shown in a six-month study to both reduce occupational stress and support the health and quality of life for the participants receiving the supplementation. *(For more information, see Appendix B for Dr. June's supplement guide.)*

- Essential oil therapy can reduce stress, alleviate anxiety, support sleep, and create a healthy and healing environment, both at home and, for many, at work too.

  - They are often used individually, but they can be mixed into combination formulas.

    - Commonly used oils to support stress reduction are bergamot, lavender, clary sage, and ylang-ylang.

    - A few words of caution regarding use of essential oils: For topical use, it is best to dilute them in a carrier oil, such as walnut or coconut. If your home has pets, choose carefully which essential oils you use in a diffuser.

Sleep Hygiene. Structuring your sleep allows your body to get into a rhythm. The goal is to support your body's natural circadian rhythm because during sleep, your body repairs and regenerates itself. The quality of sleep, not the quantity, is most important.

Here are some tips:

- Structure a sleep/wake schedule.

  - Create and follow a nightly routine. I refer to this as the *power-down hour.* Turn off electronic devices: smartphones, tablets, smartwatches, and so on. Dim the lights and slow down. This allows your natural melatonin to do its job.

- Cultivate a sacred sleep space—your bedroom.

- Choose comfortable clothing (or none) and bedding. Make sure your space has low lighting (no lighting is preferred), low noise, minimal electronics (if any), and a cooler temperature (between sixty-five and seventy degrees works for most people).

- Daily habits impact your sleep.

  - Avoid caffeine, alcohol, heavy meals, and exercise in the evening.

  - Include morning sunlight exposure, early/mid-day exercise, and consume all daily calories by six in the evening.

- Supplements can support sleep.

  - Melatonin lowers our stress hormone, cortisol, and provides potent antioxidant and anti-inflammatory properties, which support restoration and repair.

  - Magnesium promotes muscle relaxation and has calming effects, yet it is significantly depleted under prolonged stress.

  - "Tranquility" is an herbal blend supplement I commonly recommend be taken before bed. This herbal blend consists of magnolia, phellodendron, chamomile, lemon balm, oat straw, skullcap, passionflower, hops, valerian, and L-theanine.

(For more information, see Appendix B for Dr. June's supplement guide.)

Unplug and power off to recharge yourself. In today's world, we are surrounded by electromagnetic fields (EMFs). Emitted from powerlines, smart meters, computer devices, cell phones, televisions, radios, and telephones—EMFs impact people differently.

- Remember: our body weight, body mass index, bone density, hydration, and electrolyte status can alter the conductivity of, and biological reactivity to, EMFs. This is why EMFs impact people differently.

- EMFs need to be viewed like any other environmental toxin. The less exposure, the better. This is especially true now, as there has been very little research on new technology (e.g., 5G), investigating the risks it may have to human health and the environment.

- For those of you interested in the topic of EMFs and their impact on your health, I recommend a book by Nicole Bijlsman, ND, titled *Healthy Home, Healthy Family*.

Commune with nature, pets, and positive people. It's no secret that nature nurtures. Spending just 120 minutes outside every week has been associated with good health and well-being. Nature is not selective; the results of spending time in nature were consistent across key groups of individuals, including older adults and those with long-term health issues. Looking further, nature is full of microbes (the environmental microbiome), not all of which are bad, and spending more time in nature's microbiome can affect our human microbiome, improving our health. So, let's get outside and play in the dirt!

- Pets offer love and companionship, improving the quality of life for many, yet could our pet also be a probiotic? Epidemiological studies show that children growing up in households with dogs have a lower risk for developing autoimmune illnesses like asthma and allergies—and it may be related to the diversity of microbes these animals bring inside our homes.

- Selectively choosing to surround ourselves with healthy social connections not only gives us pleasure, but also influences our long-term health in ways every bit as powerful as adequate sleep, a healthy diet, and not smoking. Hundreds of studies have shown that people who have social support from family, friends, and their community are happier, have fewer health problems, and live longer.

Environment

Breathe clean air. Filtering the indoor air of your home or workspace with a high-efficiency particulate arresting (HEPA) filter is simply the smart thing to do. Placing a HEPA filter in the areas you spend most of your time (bedroom, living room, or office) helps reduce your exposure to airborne toxins such as dust mites, mold spores, pollen, and pet dander. Here are some other ways to improve the air at home:

- Although they may smell nice, replace your air fresheners and candles with natural, diffused essential oils.

  - Fragrances used in air fresheners and candles (along with almost anything else with added fragrances) release toxins such as phthalates and VCOs, along with benzene and formaldehyde (both of which are known to be carcinogenic).

  - Diffusion of essential oils (EO) provides the pleasant aroma we seek without the toxic chemicals. Please note: Although EOs are thought to be safe for humans, there are concerns of toxicity for pets. Specific EOs such as tea tree, citrus, peppermint, cinnamon, and pine (among others) are potentially toxic to both dogs and cats. Please use EOs with caution in homes with pets.[70]

- Aside from their pleasant aroma, the active components of many diffused essential oils effectively destroy several bacterial, fungal, and viral pathogens, thus potentially cleansing the very air we breathe.

Drink clean, filtered water. Filtering your water provides you with a layer of protection against the ingestion of a variety of potential chemicals, and contaminants, but which water filter is best?

- The least expensive are activated carbon filters (e.g., the Brita Filter), but effectiveness significantly varies based upon the flow rate through the filter. Some are designed to improve taste by removing chlorine and odor, while others can reduce the levels of contaminants such as asbestos, lead, mercury, and VOCs.

- The most effective filters employ a reverse osmosis system with both carbon and sediment filters. They effectively remove contaminants as carbon filters do, and they remove arsenic, fluoride, hexavalent chromium, nitrates, and perchlorate.

- A great resource tool to evaluate the health status of your home or workplace water supply is available at the Environmental Working Groups website, www.ewg.org.

Say goodbye to plastics. The convenience of plastic is what makes it challenging to give up, yet your long-term health depends on it. Plastics contain phthalates and BPA, both known to be endocrine disrupting chemicals (EDCs) and are highly toxic, even in small doses. Move toward using items made from other materials:

- Glass
- Stainless steel
- Silicone
- Ceramic
- Wood

These options provide a much safer alternative for both you and our environment. Bottom line: any time you reach for something and it's either plastic or covered in plastic (e.g., a bottle, bag, storage container, storage wrap, cutting board, kitchen utensils) ask yourself: *Is there a safer alternative?*

Review the safety rating of your personal care and beauty products. On average, women use twelve personal-care products a day, exposing themselves to 168 chemical ingredients! Men, on average, use six products, exposing themselves to 85 chemicals.[71]

- To determine how your personal care products rank on the healthy versus toxic scale, visit ewg.org/skindeep/contents/users-guide/ and find out.

- This website is packed with important health information about the personal care products you and your family may be using every day. You can use this resource to look for specific products, ingredients, and even specific companies. Additionally, you can search for cleaner and safer alternatives.

Go green to clean. Use nontoxic household products. Cleaning product labels often do not provide enough information about their ingredients to allow us to make an informed decision as to whether the product is hazardous to our health. We need to become more proactive consumers by doing our own research.

- To determine the health and safety of your household cleaning products, visit ewg.org/guides/cleaners/. Replacing your toxic products with cleaner and safer alternatives lessens your exposure and decreases your overall toxic body burden.

- If you choose to take it one step further, visit ewg.org/healthyhomeguide/ for additional tips on how to avoid health-harming chemicals at home.

Harnessing Your Habits

Eliminate all tobacco, including e-cigarettes and vaping. There is no way around this one. Tobacco is detrimental to your mouth, throat, esophagus, trachea, and lungs, as well as to your gut microbiome. It is dangerous to your overall health.

- There is no such thing as a healthy tobacco product, *including* the noncigarette alternatives.

- Quitting is the only way to decrease your risk of tobacco-related health problems. If you are a user of tobacco products, seek out the support necessary to quit. It's the single best thing you can do to improve your overall heath.

Limit alcohol consumption. To reduce the risk of alcohol-related harm, the 2015–2020 U.S. Dietary Guidelines for Americans recommends that if alcohol is consumed, it should be consumed in moderation—up to one drink per day for women and two drinks per day for men.[72]

- Now, each of us is unique in terms of our nutrient status, gut health, and genetics, but the research is clear—less is always better when it comes to the ingestion of alcohol. No matter how we attempt to frame it, alcohol is toxic to our body, and it does inhibit our estrogen metabolism and detoxification.

- Supplementation with a good-quality multivitamin and methylated B-Complex vitamin is recommended for those who consume alcohol.

Modifying cannabis use. I am a proponent of medicinal marijuana use, as it provides a valuable treatment alternative for seizure disorders, chronic pain, nausea and vomiting due to chemotherapy, and multiple sclerosis. It is currently being evaluated for the treatment of several other medical conditions as well.

- Recreational use of cannabis is a different story. Marijuana may pose problems with hormone balance in long-term, chronic users. With long-term use, the THC in marijuana induces a sustained elevated cortisol level (our body's stress hormone), suppresses thyroid function, and interferes with FSH and LH release and function, resulting in irregular or anovulatory menstrual cycles.

  - When a menstruating woman does not ovulate during her cycle, she does not produce the necessary progesterone to balance out her estrogens. The end result is that it contributes to estrogen dominance and difficulty with fertility.

  - In men, chronic consumption of THC lowers testosterone levels and sperm count and decreases sperm motility, potentially negatively impacting fertility.

- The good news, fortunately, is that after stopping long-term, chronic use, our body can restore normal function mitigating these effects.[73]

Replace your evening snacking. Our body uses the food we eat differently, depending on the time of day we consume it. This is because our insulin is more sensitive and works more efficiently in the morning and afternoon, compared to how it works in the evening and at night. Calories consumed earlier in the day are burned as fuel by the body, while calories consumed in the evening are converted to fatty acids. This means that, more than likely, they'll be stored as fat, due to more insulin resistance in the evening hours. Here are some simple ways to curb evening snacking:

- Check in with yourself to determine why you're snacking:

  Are you actually hungry?

Are you bored?

Are you tired and looking for a pick me up?

Are you sad or depressed, possibly due to low serotonin levels?

Are you lonely?

Are you irritable or angry?

It is important to figure out the reason in order to address the underlying cause.

- Substitute your snacking with hydration. Water or herbal tea may help to curb your appetite, reduce your cravings, and boost your sense of well-being.

- Establish a new evening routine or activity other than television, movies, or computer screen time. Find what suits you. Maybe it's a hot bath, journaling, drawing, coloring, listening to music, reading, quality time with loved ones, puzzles, games, cleaning, stretching, or yoga. This list is endless. It is all about replacing the habit of evening snacking with something that is good for you.

Consume your caffeine before two in the afternoon. Caffeine is almost completely metabolized through our liver; thus the health of our liver (and our genetics) impacts our ability to excrete caffeine. Why are our genetics important? Well, genetic variation in our CYP1A1 gene determines if we are a fast or a slow metabolizer of caffeine. Slow metabolizers will be more sensitive to the effects of caffeine. Keep in mind this CYP1A1 gene also plays a significant role in estrogen metabolism as well.[74]

- According to the FDA, up to 350 mg daily is considered safe for the average adult (for reference: an eight-ounce drip coffee contains about 150 mg of caffeine, variable depending on the coffee).[75]

- On average, the half-life of caffeine is five hours, which means half of the caffeine from the coffee or tea we drank at seven in the morning is still in our system at one in the afternoon. Yet how many of us reach for a pick-me-up in the afternoon containing more caffeine? Whatever it is (coffee, tea, chocolate, an energy drink), it's a good idea to not consume any after two in the afternoon.

- Accumulating caffeine can lead to hypothalamic-pituitary-adrenal axis dysregulation (HPA axis), disturbing our sleep cycle, blood sugar levels, energy levels, and overall hormone balance.

- Some lower caffeine alternatives you might consider are black, green, or white tea and decaffeinated coffee or tea. (Be careful, though. Many contaminants are often used during the decaffeination process.)

- There are some noncaffeine options as well. Water or herbal teas support overall hydration and may serve as a natural energy booster. Licorice tea, in particular, supports our HPA axis and energy levels naturally by modulating cortisol levels.

- The most impactful thing is to listen to your body. Some of us metabolize caffeine more quickly than others. If you are consuming caffeine and are experiencing challenges with anxiety, restlessness, sleep difficulty, low energy or digestive issues or suspect hormone imbalance, consider weaning off caffeine to evaluate your body's response.

Manage your medications wisely. As a naturopathic doctor, I operate with the premise of using food first, then supplementation, and then medication. However, I do agree that there are times when the best treatment for a given person may, indeed, be medication. What I do not agree with is the lack of information provided to people receiving and taking medication.

- The common acute side effects (e.g., dizziness with a new blood pressure medicine or anxiety with a new antidepressant medicine) are usually addressed. However, the silent side effects almost never are. What are silent side effects? I call them *medication-induced nutritional deficiencies*. Medications deplete nutrients over time, and these vitamin and mineral deficiencies can lead to impaired cell, tissue, and organ function.

- I provide my patients with a drug-nutrient evaluation. We discuss the validity of their medications, the short- and long-term side effects, and we replenish depleted nutrients. For those of you taking medications—prescription or over the counter—I would advise you to seek some guidance from either a naturopathic doctor, or a functional medicine or integrative practitioner to support you in this endeavor. Your long-term health will benefit.

Home in on your hobbies. I highly encourage my patients to engage in their hobbies. As a matter of fact, the intake forms I use in my practice ask my patients to list their hobbies and how often they engage in them. Why? Because hobbies are important, providing intermittent periods of creativity, joy, fun, physical exercise, or relaxation.

Hobbies have a way of helping balance our lives by making the stressors of work and life more tolerable. When the hobbies section of the intake form is left blank, I take the time to ask why it was left blank. Everyone seems to have hobbies, yet the two most common responses I hear when it comes to why they aren't currently enjoying them are *I don't have the time* and *I don't have the energy*.

Despite the many positive aspects of hobbies, there can be health risks associated with them. I ask you to consider taking some time to evaluate potential exposures you may be coming into contact with while partaking in your hobbies. Here are a few things to consider:

- Seek and use less toxic, safer products and materials whenever possible.

- Use the correct and effective personal protective equipment or safety equipment.

- Appropriately clean and store items, equipment, and materials.

- Always have a clean source of air to breathe.

Chapter 7

Liberate Your Lymphatics

Twelve Ways to "Liberate Your Lymphatics"

1. Exercise and Movement—Just Do It!

Walking is simple and safe, and just thirty minutes a day significantly improves lymphatic function by decreasing the accumulation of inflammatory cells within the lymphatics and the leakiness of the lymphatic vessels and enhancing gene expression in lymphatic endothelial cells. Rebounding on a mini trampoline is a superior way to move your lymph. In fact, research done by NASA found rebounding exercise to be 68 percent more efficient that jogging as a total body exercise.[76]

Yoga increases lymph flow, too, and relieves lymphatic congestion in unique ways: First, the rhythmical tensing and relaxing of the muscles during yoga poses facilitates lymph flow. Second, inversion poses, such as legs up the wall or shoulder stands, reverse the effects of gravity to enhance lymph drainage. And third, yoga's emphasis on conscious breathing (*pranayama*) is a lymphatic pump in and of itself, helping direct lymph flow through the deep channels and ducts within the abdomen and chest. I would take it one step further and add that incorporating other TCM practices, such as Tai Qi and Qi Gong, would be excellent lymphatic movers as well.

2. Hydration

Dehydration contributes to thicken lymph, hindering its flow through the lymphatic vessels. Hydration promotes lymph flow by reducing the viscosity of lymph fluid. Work toward consuming half of your body weight in ounces of clean, filtered water daily.

A few additional pearls of wisdom:

- Herbal teas, unlike black, green, or white teas, do not contain caffeine and therefore support hydration. Please note that despite not containing caffeine, some herbal teas, such as parsley, dandelion, horsetail, and hibiscus tea, have diuretic properties and may contribute to dehydration if consumed in large amounts.

- Drinking smaller amounts of liquid at more frequent intervals is better absorbed than larger volumes all at one time.

- Adding minerals or electrolytes, in the form of drops or powders, to your filtered water results in enhanced uptake into cells, promoting better cellular hydration.

3. Diet

Diets high in sugar, artificial and processed foods, animal products, dairy products, eggs, refined carbohydrates, soda, and coffee distort gut function, triggering systemic inflammation. Inflammation leads to congestion and swelling, therefore inhibiting the flow of lymph and other bodily fluids. Diets high in anti-inflammatory plant-based foods reduce inflammation and promote lymph flow. They include:

- Vegetables (dandelion greens, arugula, watercress)
- Citrus fruits
- Avocados
- Beans

- Sprouts
- Figs
- Some whole grains (oats, quinoa, buckwheat, millet)
- Some oils (avocado, olive, coconut, fish, and flax)
- Some herbs and spices (turmeric, ginger, rosemary, and cinnamon)

4. Sleep

Unlike the rest of our body, our central nervous system (CNS) lacks conventional lymphatic vessels. Instead, the CNS must rely on what is known as the glymphatic system. Unlike our lymphatic system, which relies on movement and contractions to function, our glymphatic system is activated only during sleep. Therefore, quality sleep is critical for our brain to drain and cleanse itself of neurotoxic waste products produced during our waking hours.

Make sleep a priority and strive for good sleep hygiene practices. Here are my top recommendations:

- Establish a set sleep schedule, even on the weekends, striving for seven to eight hours a night.

- Create a *power-down hour* by turning off all electronics (e.g., cell phones, iPads, computers, monitors) and dimming lights one hour prior to bedtime to allow your own melatonin to do its job.

- Start your day by getting outside in the natural sunlight. Not only does this activate your brain, but it also balances your circadian rhythm by increasing the production of serotonin, and eventually melatonin, to enhance your sleep cycle.

- Have a gratitude moment before sleep. This can be done by yourself or with your loved ones.

5. Stress Reduction

The susceptibility to stress varies from person to person because it is influenced by many factors. Our genetic vulnerability, coping style, personality type, and social support system all impact our susceptibility to stress. It is clear chronic stress is a severe medical concern, as estimates show that 75 to 90 percent of all visits to primary care physicians are for stress-related problems.[77]

Chronic stress contributes to a state of sympathetic nervous system (SNS) dominance, resulting in vasoconstriction, reduced blood flow, reduced lymphatic function, digestive dysfunction, systemic inflammation, and impaired immune system function directly contributing to hormone imbalance and all illness seen today. Here are my top three tips for reducing stress:

- Deep-breathing exercises dispersed throughout your day cost nothing, require minimal time and effort, and can be done absolutely anywhere!

- Physical exercise stimulates the release of brain endorphins and neurotransmitters, which is proven to support sleep, mood, and stress reduction. Keep in mind that even short intervals of exercise count.

- Practice mindfulness. Being present and focused on the here and now limits the brain from unnecessary distractions, reducing stress hormone, anxiety, and depression.

6. Limit Restrictive Clothing

Lymphatic flow is somewhat restricted in areas of our body simply due to our anatomy. Areas where natural bending occurs, such as the ankle, behind the knee, the groin, the waist, the axilla (armpit), and the elbow, are more prone to obstructed lymph flow. Enhancing lymphatic flow is the goal, so limiting prolonged sitting, sitting cross-legged, and wearing tight-fitting clothing (especially those leaving an indentation) at your ankles, wrists, chest, and waist can be helpful. Also, breast tissue is rich with lymphatics, and a constricting bra will impede lymph flow and drainage.

7. Dry Skin Brushing

Usually done before showering using a natural, soft-bristled brush, the mechanical action of this do-it-yourself technique promotes lymph flow and circulation by gently brushing your skin in the same direction as the lymph is traveling—starting at your feet and hands and moving upward toward your collarbone. In addition, the natural process of skin exfoliation is enhanced by dry brushing, promoting detoxification and revealing the healthy new skin underneath.

8. Lymphatic Massage

Manual lymphatic drainage technique is a type of massage using a very light, superficial massage with gentle, rhythmic skin distention. The strokes feel more like a sweeping or brushing motion and are designed to decongest lymph nodes and facilitate the flow of lymph from the periphery tissues back toward the heart. This massage can be self-administered as well as done by a trained professional.

9. Hydrotherapy

Hydrotherapy, (also known as *Water Cure*) is the use of water, externally or internally, in any of its forms (water, ice, steam) to promote health and treat disease. It has been used widely in ancient cultures, dating as far back as the eighteenth century. The beauty is that many hydrotherapy treatments can be applied at home, are cost-effective and convenient, and foster self-care. Hydrotherapy can be a valuable adjunctive therapy for both acute and chronic conditions.

Hydrotherapy utilizes the contrasting water temperatures, hot and cold, to stimulate blood flow within the digestive tract, facilitate lymphatic flow, enhance immune function, and balance the sympathetic (fight or flight) and parasympathetic (rest and repair) nervous systems, all of which are essential to restoring and maintaining hormone balance within our body. Two easy home therapies include:

A. **Contrasting foot bath**. Best done before bed due to its relaxing properties. You'll use two basins—one filled with hot water (to tolerance) and one cold (to tolerance). Start by soaking your feet for three minutes in the hot water, then soaking your feet in the cold water for thirty seconds. Repeat this process for three cycles, always ending with the cold water. Dry your feet well and retire for the night.

B. **Contrasting shower**. There are two options for this one. You can either end your shower with thirty seconds of cool or cold water, or you can end your shower by alternating between warm and cool water for up to three cycles (always ending with cold water).

You will need to take precautions if you have a decreased sensitivity to hot and cold, are pregnant, or have an acute injury. I recommend checking with your provider.

10. Sauna Therapy (Medical Grade Far Infrared Sauna)

Not only does it feel good, but sauna therapy also provides many medicinal benefits. Sitting in a hot sauna raises our body's core temperature, induces sweating, and is a safe and gentle means of mobilizing fat-soluble xenobiotics, toxic chemicals, and heavy metals. Sweating during sauna therapy reduces overall fluid levels in our blood, making it easier for our lymphatics to pick up the toxin-rich intercellular fluid and return it to our circulation for elimination via our kidneys, liver, and bowel.

Hydration is important to maximize the benefits of sauna therapy, so be sure to hydrate before and replenish after each session with electrolyte-rich fluids. Electrolytes and minerals are lost in sweat.

Temperature, duration, and frequency of sauna therapy are unique for each person. Many factors can impact your tolerance to sauna therapy. Taking into account your overall vitality is an important consideration. One question I ask all my patients before initiating sauna therapy is: *How easily does your body sweat?* This is helpful in determining the starting temperature and duration of the initial treatments.

As with most treatments, some potential contraindications may exist. Check with your provider before using any sauna if you have a heart arrhythmia, hypertension, obstructive lung disease, diabetes, or are pregnant. Some general guidelines for sauna therapy include:

- **Temperature**: For most people, the range is somewhere between 110 and 130 degrees Fahrenheit. Starting low and working up is best, and for most, 110 degrees is a safe starting point. If you find your body begins to sweat after five minutes and is sweating heavily by ten minutes, that temperature is right for you. If not, increase the temperature by five to ten degrees during your next session. The goal is to find the temperature that is right for you. I have found that engaging in some exercise, like a brisk ten-minute walk, prior to getting into the sauna induces perspiring more quickly. I recommend this to my patients as well, so they are able to maximize their sauna sessions.

- **Duration**: The initial session is usually fifteen minutes at 110 degrees. Once you find your optimal temperature as mentioned above, the goal is to work up to thirty minutes of full sweating.

- **Frequency**: Because the metabolic effects of sauna therapy mimic that of exercise, adequate rest between sessions is needed to allow for healing to occur. It is important to listen to your body. For most people, three to five times a week is best. That's why having a sauna in your home would allow you the greatest ease and flexibility with timing your sessions. As with any treatment, it is important to listen to your body and talk with your healthcare provider for additional guidance.

11. Lymphagogues

Lymphagogues are herbal medicines that support your lymphatics. Using plants as medicine for healing is as old as humankind itself. Herbal medicine, also known as *botanical medicine*, refers to the use of a plant's seeds, roots, flowers, leaves, bark, or fruit for medicinal purposes. Plants are powerful medicine with very few side effects compared to pharmaceutical drugs. The beauty of herbal medicine is that one plant can have multiple active constituents and impact many body systems, as well as treat multiple conditions. For example, let's look at the medicinal benefits of the dandelion plant.

The bitter nature of dandelion root stimulates secretion of gastric acid from the stomach, bile from the gallbladder, and liver and pancreatic enzymes from the pancreas, making it an amazing herb for a variety of digestive issues, as well as female menstrual cycle issues. The leaf inhibits sodium reabsorption, providing a diuretic effect, thus useful for lowering blood pressure or reducing edema. Dandelion also possesses antiplatelet aggregation properties (which makes our blood less sticky), reducing the risk for blood clotting, thus useful for cardiovascular health and blood sugar support.

It is important to note that herbs may interact with medications, and for this reason it's essential to have an expert clinician evaluate everything you're taking, including pharmaceuticals, OTCs, and dietary supplements. I recommend you work with a naturopathic doctor to find the best combination of herbs for your specific needs.

Blending herbs together in the form of an herbal tincture is one of the oldest and most common delivery methods. Herbs shown to promote lymphatic flow, of which there are many, are known as lymphagogues. I'll share some of my favorites:

Lymphagogues for breast and upper body drainage:

- *Phytolacca americana* (Poke root)

- *Trifolium pratense* (Red clover)

- *Galium aparine* (Cleavers)

- *Scrophularia nodosa* (Figwort)

- *Echinacea purpurea* (Echinacea)

- *Baptisia tinctoria* (Wild indigo root)

Lymphagogues with antimicrobial properties (for gut health):

- *Arctium lappa* (Burdock root)

- *Mahonia aquifolium* (Oregon grape root)

- *Coptis chinensis* (Golden thread)

- *Hydrastis canadensis* (Goldenseal)

Lymphagogues with cholagogue properties (for lymph flow, gallbladder, and liver health):

- *Arctium lappa* (Burdock root)

- *Mahonia aquifolium* (Oregon grape root)

- *Taraxacum officinale* (Dandelion root)

- *Coptis chinensis* (Golden thread)

- *Hydrastis canadensis* (Goldenseal)

12. Homeopathic Drainage Remedies

Homeopathy, otherwise known as *homeopathic medicine*, dates back to the late eighteenth century. Founded by Samuel Hahnemann, a German physician, this form of gentle, yet powerful alternative medicine uses extremely diluted amounts of specific natural substances (plant, mineral, or animal) to treat various ailments.

Often thought of as one and the same, drainage and detoxification are two separate processes in the body. For our body to successfully detoxify, the drainage pathways must be open and flowing; otherwise toxicity and disease set in. Homeopathic drainage remedies aid in opening the emunctories (or organs of eliminations—lymph, liver, lung, kidney, gastrointestinal tract, skin, and mucus membranes) to assist the body with its normal and natural physiologic drainage processes to promote detoxification and elimination of waste.

Due to the complexity involved with choosing and using homeopathic drainage remedies, seeking guidance from a trained homeopathic or naturopathic doctor would be best.

Chapter 8

Build Your Bile

7 Ways To "Build Your Bile"

1. Diet

Bitters—a digestive aide that blends plant tinctures—are best! They stimulate digestive secretions from the stomach, gallbladder, liver, and pancreas, promoting digestion and detoxification. Get away from the sauces, dips, dollops, and condiments and back to using plants, herbs, and spices. But remember, food is medicine, and when it comes to bitters, a small amount packs a powerful punch.

Here's a health tip: Ten minutes before eating, take 1 teaspoon of apple cider vinegar or lemon juice in a half-ounce of water to naturally stimulate digestion. (Use caution if you have active GERD or gastritis.) To gain even greater effect, limit liquid intake with meals to prevent diluting your digestive secretions.

Bitter Foods:

- Dandelion greens
- Arugula
- Watercress
- Kale
- Radicchio
- Bitter melon
- Endive

Bitter Herbs and Spices:

- Dill
- Parsley
- Thyme
- Oregano
- Mint
- Ginger
- Cinnamon
- Coriander
- Caraway
- Turmeric

It's a good idea to focus on healthy fats, too. Some healthy fats are:

- Omega-3 (found in sardines, anchovies, salmon, flaxseed, chia seed, walnuts)

- Omega-6 (hemp seeds, sunflower seeds, pumpkin seeds, pine nuts, pistachios)

- Omega-7 (found in macadamia nuts, avocado, olives, and their oil)

Also be sure to fill up on fiber! Fiber feeds your gut flora and facilitates gut motility. The daily recommendation is 30 to 40 grams (from food, not supplements), yet the average adult intake in the U.S. is only 15 grams a day.[78] Fiber is found only in plants, not in animal products. And we need both soluble fiber (absorbs water during digestion) and insoluble fiber (remains unchanged during digestion) in our daily diet to maximize gut health. (*See Table # 1 below for a high-fiber foods list.*)

Consuming choline-rich foods is important, too. Choline is an essential nutrient needed for your body's production of *phosphatidylcholine* (PC), a major component of every cell membrane, and a key component of bile. PC is what keeps our bile thin and slippery, allowing for smooth bile flow, ultimately enhancing fat absorption and hormone and waste elimination.

It is important to note there is evidence to support that as much as 50 percent of the U.S. population carries genetic variations (an SNP in their PEMT gene), making it necessary for them to consume even higher amounts of choline greater than the recommended average daily nutrient intake, or adequate intake (AI): 425 mg a day for women, 450 mg a day for pregnant women, 550 mg a day for lactating women, and 550 mg a day for men.[79]

Choline food sources (*see Table # 2 below for more complete list*):

- Animals: eggs, pork, beef, fish (salmon), shellfish (scallops and mollusks), and turkey

- Plants: artichokes, Brussels sprouts, leafy greens (collards, beet greens, and Swiss chard), beans (pink and black), seeds (sunflower and pumpkin), quinoa

2. Hydrate, Hydrate, Hydrate

Keeping hydrated is critical, as our bile is nearly 95 percent water. Strive to drink half your body weight in ounces (for example, 150 pounds body weight = 75 ounces) of water and herbal teas (these do not contain caffeine) per day.

Drinking your liquids between meals is best to prevent diluting your natural stomach acid while eating. Start your day with one tablespoon lemon juice in 8 ounces of warm water. Drinking lemon water when you wake up enhances digestion and bile flow due to its natural, bitter properties.

3. Movement Is Medicine

Consistent exercise reduces the risk for obesity and elevated cholesterol, both significant risk factors for gallstone formation and gallbladder disease. Elevated body mass index (BMI) and increased abdominal fat mass may contribute to gallbladder hypomotility (decreased contraction of the gallbladder) and bile stasis (efficient bile flow), particularly in women.

A med-analysis review article published July 2016 in the *Journal of Physical Activity and Health* concluded that regular physical exercise, vigorous and nonvigorous, lowered the risk of gallbladder disease regardless of the person's body mass index (BMI).[80]

The solution is using movement as your medicine. Strive to achieve at least the current exercise recommendation (a total of 150 minutes of moderate to intense activity, or 75 minutes of vigorous intense activity, every week). The key to your success is choosing activities you enjoy and consistently engaging (even in short intervals—ten minutes at a time) makes a significant difference over time.

In a 2016 study of type 2 diabetic people, researchers from the University of Otago in New Zealand discovered that timed-interval walking—a brisk ten-minute walk following each meal—rather than a thirty-minute walk every day, had a more profound impact on blood sugar, resulting in a 12 percent reduction.[81]

4. Sleep

Sleep is our body's most potent natural antioxidant and anti-inflammatory. During sleep, our body is repairing, replenishing, and rejuvenating itself. So, if you're not sleeping well (falling and staying asleep, along with waking feeling refreshed), you're at greater risk for illness and disease.

If you are not sleeping well, take a detailed self-inventory and seek help from a doctor as needed in order to find the underlying cause (or causes). Causes vary from physical disturbance (pain), medical issues (hormone imbalance, gastroesophageal reflux), psychological conditions (stress, depression, or anxiety), and environmental issues (bright light, pets on the bed, others' snoring). Chronic sleep disturbance leads to altered hormone regulation, elevated inflammation, weight gain, and impaired gut function.

One of the more common and under-recognized causes of impaired sleep is sleep apnea. It is estimated that 22 million Americans suffer from sleep apnea, with 80 percent of moderate to severe obstructive sleep apnea (OSA) cases being undiagnosed. Surprisingly, OSA can strike people of any age, including infants and children, yet is most commonly seen in overweight and obese individuals.

The hypoxia (low oxygen state) associated with OSA may lead to an increase in fat accumulation in the liver, causing nonalcoholic fatty liver disease (NAFLD) or hepatic inflammation, which we have more recently learned contributes to impaired gallbladder motility, decreased bile flow, and gallstone formation.

5. Stress Reduction

Reducing stress balances our sympathetic nervous system response (fight or flight) with our parasympathetic nervous system response (rest and digest). We have all heard chronic stress negatively impacts our overall health, yet were you aware that chronic stress can impair your gallbladder function? Chronic social stress has shown to result in both gallbladder hypertrophy (enlargement) and bile retention due to inhibition of gallbladder emptying.[82] Much like exercise, finding the stress reduction techniques that resonate most with you and building them into your daily life are keys to long-term success and health.

6. Herbal Medicine

Using herbal medicine means utilizing the power of plants to produce and move bile. Medicinal herbs used to stimulate digestive secretions are known as *bitters*. Those used to stimulate bile flow are known as cholagogues (bile movers). And herbs used to stimulate bile production are known as choleretics (bile makers).

The following list contains several of the more commonly used botanicals, some used alone, yet most often used in various combinations, to support digestive health and bile flow and gallbladder and liver function. Most often they are taken before meals:

- Gentian (*Gentian lutea*)
- Oregon grape root and barberry (*Mahonia spp.*)
- Celandine (*Chelidonium majus*)
- Burdock root (*Arctium lappa*)
- Yellow dock (*Achillea millefolium*)
- Dandelion root (*Taraxacum officinalis*)
- Goldenseal (*Hydrastis canadensis*)
- Artichoke leaf extract (*Cynara scolymus*)
- Ginger (*Zingiber officinalis*)
- Rhubarb (*Rheum officinalis*)
- Rosemary (*Rosmarinus officinalis*)
- Turmeric (*Curcuma longa*)
- Peppermint (*Mentha piperita*)

Please note that herbal medicine is powerful medicine and may be contraindicated in some conditions or with some medications. Seek the guidance from a naturopathic doctor or another qualified, licensed professional to achieve your safest and best outcome.

7. Supplementation

In clinical practice, I always address my patients' digestive health first. I start with using digestive bitters and bowel binders. Why? Because the goal is to enhance gastric secretions and keep the digestive track moving. Bitters stimulate the movement of bile through the liver and gallbladder and into the small intestine. Bile serves as a carrier for hormones, waste materials, and toxicants needing to get out of the body. I add binders to prevent the recirculation of these waste materials by grabbing and holding onto them in the bowel and escorting them out in stool. For best results with supplementation, consult with a naturopathic doctor or qualified, licensed professional.

Bitter formulas are a combination of herbs, spices, and, at times, essential oils taken before meals to stimulate digestive secretions. They may be in the form of capsules or, most often, liquid tinctures. My favorite combination contains gentian, dandelion, ginger, turmeric, artichoke, and anise.

Three certified-organic, commercially available bitter tincture products include:

- Bittersweet Elixir by Wise Woman Herbals
- Sweetish Bitters by Gaia Herbs
- Better Bitters Classic by Herb Pharm

Binders are insoluble particles that are able to pass through our gut unabsorbed, yet they have the ability to tightly bind numerous toxins. Once bound, these toxins (pesticides, herbicides, chemicals, metals, bacterial metabolites, hormones, xenoestrogens, and endotoxins) can safely be excreted through our stool, reducing the overall toxic load on our body.

Binders are available in powder, capsule, or liquid form. For best results, binders are taken about thirty to sixty minutes after meals.

Everyone's digestive tract is unique, so some binders may cause more gas, bloating, and constipation than others. Always start with a low dose and work up.

Binders are either positively or negatively charged; therefore, different binders have an affinity for different toxins. They may be taken as an individual supplement or in a combination product.

Common individual binding agents include:

- Activated charcoal – for pesticides, herbicides, molds, persistent organic pollutants, volatile organic compounds, and binding endotoxins (or LPS) in the gut

- Bentonite clay – for mycotoxins and aflatoxins from mold and food, organochlorine pesticides, and metals like lead, cadmium, and copper

- Chlorella – for heavy metals, particularly mercury

- Modified citrus pectin and alginates – for heavy metals, pesticides, radioactive particles, and other toxins

- Zeolite – for metals, ammonia, mycotoxins, and aflatoxins

Quality commercially available combination products:

- GI Detox by Bio-Botanical Research, Inc
- Ultra Binder by Quicksilver Scientific
- PectaClear Detox Formula by EcoNugenics
- ZeoBind by BioPure

Phosphatidylcholine (PC) functions to protect the liver, reduce gallstone formation, and keep bile thin and slippery for smoother flow and easier detoxification.

I am a firm believer in using food first whenever possible, and a diet rich in choline may negate the need for supplementation with PC. (*See Table #2 Below for a list of choline rich foods.*) When necessary, PC is available in powder, liquid, and capsule form and is taken before meals.

Who may benefit from PC supplementation?

- Individuals who are sensitive to bitters. If PC is taken before meals, it may be a helpful alternative to enhance bile flow.

- Those living a vegan, vegetarian, or carbo-tarian lifestyle, since obtaining enough dietary choline may be more difficult. Low choline can lead to deficient PC.

- Those with genetic polymorphisms in their PEMT gene. This gene is responsible for making PC in limited amounts when choline intake in the diet is insufficient.

- Those with a genetic polymorphism in their MTHFR gene. Too little folate in your body can drive up the demand for more choline.

- Postmenopausal women. Estrogen supports the function of the PEMT gene and choline production.

- Pregnant or breastfeeding women. The demand for choline is significantly increased during these times.

Ox Bile is derived from oxen (commonly adult male cattle or bovines) and is especially helpful for those who have had their gallbladder removed in order to replace deficient bile.

Ox bile is taken prior to meals, especially a high-fat meal, for those who cannot tolerate fats. It can be taken in capsule form by itself, or most often, as a component within a digestive enzyme formula. The dosage needed will vary. Always start low and work up, as bile has antimicrobial properties and may trigger a *Herxheimer reaction or die-off reaction.*

Lipase is an enzyme produced mainly in the pancreas and, to lesser extent, in your mouth and stomach. Lipase, with help from bile, breaks down the fats in food so they can be absorbed in the intestines. It can be taken in capsule form by itself, or most often, as a component within a digestive enzyme formula. It works best taken just prior to eating meals.

Taurine is an amino acid found almost exclusively in animal protein sources. It plays a critical role in our body's ability to synthesis healthy bile in the liver. Supplementation may be needed for those living a vegan, vegetarian, or carbo-tarian lifestyle, as obtaining enough dietary taurine may be difficult.

Best food sources for taurine:

- Fish (tuna)
- Shellfish (crab, scallops)
- Beef
- Pork
- Chicken
- Eggs
- Dairy

Alternative sources: some seaweeds are known to contain very small amounts of taurine. Red edible algae such as mafunori (*Gloiopeltis tenax*), fukurofunori (*Gloiopeltis furcata*), kabanori (*Gracilaria textorii*), and ogonori (*Gracilaria vermiculophylla*) have been found to have the highest content and may someday be used to create functional foods rich in naturally occurring taurine.

Table 1: High Fiber Food Sources:[83]

Food	Portion	Fiber (grams)
Fruit		
Avocado	1 cup, cubed	10.0
Pear	1 medium	5.5
Apple (with skin)	1 medium	4.4
Raspberries	1 cup	8.0
Blackberries	1 cup	7.6
Vegetables		
Artichoke	1 medium	10.3
Brussels sprouts	1 cup cooked	4.0
Beets	1 cup cooked	3.8
Carrot	1 cup chopped	3.6
Broccoli	1 cup chopped	2.4
Legumes		
Navy beans	1 cup cooked	19.1
Split peas	1 cup cooked	16.3
Lentils	1 cup cooked	15.6
Black beans	1 cup cooked	15.0
Chickpeas	1 cup cooked	12.6
Seeds		
Chia seeds	1 ounce	10.6
Flaxseed	1 ounce	7.6
Sesame seeds	1 ounce	3.3
Sunflower seeds	1 ounce	2.4
Pumpkin seed	1 ounce	1.1
Nuts		
Almond	1 ounce	3.4
Pistachio	1 ounce	2.9
Pecan	1 ounce	2.7
Hazelnut	1 ounce	2.7
Peanut	1 ounce	2.7

Grains		
Shredded wheat	1 cup	7.9
Bulgur	½ cup cooked	4.1
Oats	1 cup cooked	4.0
Pearled barley	½ cup cooked	3.0
Quinoa	½ cup cooked	2.6
Carbohydrates		
Sweet potato (with skin)	1 medium	3.8
Pumpkin	½ cup cooked	3.6
Popcorn (air popped)	3 cups	3.5
Parsnips	½ cup cooked	3.1
Winter squash	½ cup cooked	2.9

Table 2: Food Sources of Choline[84]

Food	Milligrams (mg) per serving	Percent DV*
Beef liver (pan fried, 3 oz)	356	65
Egg (hard boiled, 1 large egg)	147	27
Beef top round, lean (braised, 3 oz)	117	21
Soybeans (roasted, ½ cup)	107	19
Chicken breast (roasted, 3 oz)	72	13
Beef, ground, 93% lean (broiled, 3 oz)	72	13
Fish, cod, Atlantic (cooked, dry heat, 3 oz)	71	13
Potatoes, red, (baked with skin, 1 large potato)	57	10
Wheat germ (toasted, 1 oz)	51	9
Beans, kidney (canned, ½ cup)	45	8
Quinoa (cooked, 1 cup)	43	8
Milk, 1% fat (1 cup)	43	8
Yogurt, vanilla (nonfat, 1 cup)	38	7
Brussels sprouts (boiled, ½ cup)	32	6
Broccoli (chopped, boiled, drained, ½ cup)	31	6
Mushrooms, shiitake (cooked, ½ cup)	27	5

Cottage cheese (nonfat, 1 cup)	26	5
Tuna, white (canned in water, 3 oz)	25	5
Peanuts (dry roasted, ¼ cup)	24	4
Cauliflower (chopped, boiled, drained, ½ cup)	24	4
Peas, green (boiled, ½ cup)	24	4
Sunflower seeds (oil roasted, ¼ cup)	19	3
Rice, brown, long-grain (cooked, 1 cup)	19	3
Bread, pita, whole wheat (1 large piece)	17	3
Cabbage (boiled, ½ cup)	15	3
Tangerine/mandarin orange sections (½ cup)	10	2
Beans, snap (raw, ½ cup)	8	1
Kiwifruit (raw, ½ cup slice)	7	1
Carrots (raw, chopped, ½ cup)	6	1
Apples with skin (chopped ½ cup)	2	0

DV = Daily Value as developed by the U.S. Food and Drug Administration (FDA)

A Special Note About Your PEMT Gene

So, what is PEMT and why is it important?

Your PEMT gene (or *Phosphatidylethanolamine N-methyltransferase*) encodes for an enzyme that, along with help from your methylation cycle, is responsible for making what is known as *phosphatidylcholine* (PC) for your body. Unfortunately, this gene gets very little attention and is often overlooked when it comes to hormone balance. Additionally, it is estimated that up to 50 percent of the U.S. population has a genetic SNP in their PEMT gene, potentially hindering their body's ability to produce PC.

Why is this so important? Having healthy levels of PC is important for several reasons, yet when it comes to hormone balance and detoxification, the role PC plays in maintaining the health and integrity of your cell membranes, as well as building healthy bile, is what is most important.

Cell membranes must be fluid and flexible. A healthy membrane allows for easier transport of nutrients into the cell, as well as the transport for hormones, xenoestrogens, and other toxicants out of the cell. When PC is readily available, cell membranes are more fluid and flexible, facilitating easier transport and preventing intracellular toxicity. Without enough PC, hormones, xenoestrogens, and toxicants can become trapped inside your cells, which leads to intercellular toxicity.

PC plays an integral part in the production of bile. To flow smoothly and easily, bile needs to be thin and slippery, not thick and sludgy. PC helps maintain the slippery texture of bile, facilitating its flow. Since bile is the major carrier of your hormones and other toxicants, flow is the name of the game. Healthy bile and healthy bile flow are necessary to transport hormones, xenoestrogens, and toxicants out of the liver into the small intestine for eventual elimination through the bowel.

Here are three ways to support your PEMT gene to maximize PC production for healthy detoxification:

1. **Consume a diet rich in choline** (a building block for PC). Be mindful of choline deficiency if you are eating a restrictive diet, such as a vegan diet for example, since choline content is highest in animal products (*refer to choline-rich food list*).

2. **Become more aware of situations and conditions** which may stress your PEMT gene. Pregnancy and breastfeeding are great examples because, while in these conditions, your body's demand for choline significantly increases, placing additional stress on your PEMT gene.

3. **Support the health and function** of your methylation cycle as it impacts the function of your PEMT gene. A diet rich in leafy greens keeps your folate levels up. Folate, along with your B-vitamins, keeps the methylation cycle running. When your body is methylating well, the demand for choline is far less, yet if your body is not methylating well, the demand for choline rises, putting a greater strain on your PEMT gene.

Chapter 9

Love Your Liver

Supporting Your Phase 1 Estrogen Detoxification[85, 86]

Focus on food first (organic produce and organic, grass-fed animal and dairy products) by eating:

- Iron-rich foods, like meats (especially red meat), dark leafy greens, beans and lentils, blackstrap molasses. (All Phase 1 enzymes are dependent upon iron.)

- Fruits and vegetables (7–9 servings a day) that are rich in antioxidants, fiber, polyphenols and flavonoids, that promote and maintain a healthier pH balance in your body. Strive to eat all the colors of the rainbow every day.

- Cruciferous vegetables, like broccoli, cauliflower, cabbage, Brussels sprouts, kale, collards, turnips. These are best if chopped and slightly heated to maximize their medicinal effects on estrogens. They are also rich in Indol-3-carbinol (I3C), which potentiates 2-OH estrogen (safer estrogen) pathways.

- Apiaceae family of foods, like carrots, fennel, anise, cumin, celery, dill, cilantro, coriander, caraway, and parsley. These foods inhibit the 4-OH estrogen (more dangerous estrogen) pathway.

- Sulphur-rich glutathione-enhancing foods, like garlic, ginger, onions, broccoli sprouts, and eggs. These support the production of our body's most potent natural antioxidant—glutathione, which neutralizes reactive estrogen metabolites, thus protecting your DNA.

Supplements (always best to discuss first with your provider):

- Antioxidants: vitamins A, C, D and E, resveratrol, CoQ10. As with food, rotation and moderation of antioxidant supplements is best.

- Minerals: selenium, copper, zinc, iron, magnesium, manganese. Serve as co-factors supporting the function of Phase 1 and Phase 2 enzymes.

- B-vitamins: B1, B2, B3, B6, B12, and folate (B9). Serve as co-factors supporting the function of Phase 1 and Phase 2 enzymes.

- Indol-3-Carbinol (I3C) or Diindolylmethane (DIM): derived for I3C. Potentiates 2-OH estrogen (safer estrogen) pathway.

- N-Acetylcysteine: one of the building blocks for the natural production of glutathione. Aids in neutralizing reactive estrogen metabolites.

Lifestyle:

Avoid inhibitors of Phase 1 detoxification enzymes:

- This consists of smoking, drinking alcohol, eating charred meats (BBQ), and consuming high amounts of grapefruit juice.

- Also, environmental chemicals such as phthalates, BPA, PCBs, PAHs, and Xenoestrogens.

Ways to induce Phase 1 detoxification enzymes:

- Organic coffee contains caffeine, which potentiates your 2-OH estrogen (safer estrogen) pathway.

- Sleep is associated with higher levels of melatonin, one of our body's potent natural antioxidants, which regulates many metabolic processes in our body. Melatonin production in our body increases in response to darkness. The higher levels induce relaxation to promote sleep.

- Exercise enhances lymphatic flow, circulation, deep breathing, and sweating—all of which promote and enhance overall detoxification.

Supporting Your Phase 2 Estrogen Detoxification

Focus on food first (organic produce and organic, grass-fed animal and dairy products) by eating:

- Sulfur-rich foods, like cruciferous vegetables, garlic, onion, egg yolks, ginger, meat, poultry, and fish, support the natural production of glutathione, necessary to neutralize reactive estrogen metabolites.

- Broccoli sprouts are considered a super food rich in the phytonutrient *sulforaphane* that increases the natural production of glutathione and promotes the action of Phase 2 liver detoxification enzymes.

- Amino acids, like glycine, cysteine, taurine, and methionine (from meat, poultry, eggs, and nuts), are essential for the excretion of Phase 1 metabolites.

- Polyphenols, especially ellagic acid (from pomegranates, berries, walnuts, and other plants), enhance the action of

Phase 2 enzymes (promoting elimination) while reducing the action of Phase 1 enzymes (preventing the buildup of reactive estrogen metabolites)

- Flavonoids in fruits and vegetables are rich in antioxidants, fiber, polyphenols, and flavonoids. They promote and maintain a healthier pH balance in your body, so strive to eat the colors of the rainbow in your daily diet.

Supplements (always best to discuss first with your provider):

- Methyl donors: magnesium, SAMe, betaine or trimethylglycine (TMG), and choline, critical factors for Phase 2 detoxification.

- B-vitamins: B2, B5, B6, B12, and folate enhance the function of Phase 2 enzymes.

- Nfr2 Enhancers: curcumin, resveratrol, silymarin (from milk thistle), and sulforaphane. Each has the ability to upregulate our body's Nrf2 pathways, our body's innate mechanism for creating antioxidants.

- Glutathione: Liposomal form is the best absorbed when taking it in supplement form. N-Acetyl-Cysteine (NAC) is a precursor to glutathione and may be used in place of glutathione.

Lifestyle:

Avoid inhibitors of Phase 2 detoxification and use caution with:

- Environmental chemicals (phthalates, BPA, PCBs, PAHs, xenoestrogens)

- Prescription and over-the-counter medications

- Long-term, highly restrictive diets (this may lead to nutrient deficiencies)

Ways to induce Phase 2 detoxification:

- Stay active: exercise actives our Nrf2 pathways (our body's natural mechanism for creating antioxidants, known to enhance Phase 2 detoxification).

- Intermittent fasting: upregulates our Nrf2 pathways promoting detoxification.

Supporting Your Phase 2.5 Estrogen Metabolism

Focus on food first (organic produce and organic, grass-fed animal and dairy products) by eating:

- Antioxidants neutralize oxidative stress and reduce inflammation to enhance transport protein function. They are rich in vegetables and fruits. Strive to eat seven to nine servings of fruits and vegetables and the colors of the rainbow every day.

Healthy fats support the fluidity and flexibility of cell membranes.

- Omega-3s (wild-caught salmon, mackerel, and halibut and flax, chia, and hemp seeds)

- Omega-7s (macadamia nuts, sardines, anchovies)

- Monounsaturated fats (olive, avocado, nuts, seeds)

- Medium Chain Triglycerides (MTC) (coconut oil, palm kernel oil)

- Choline is a building block for phosphatidylcholine necessary to make and repair cell membranes and to build healthy bile. Rich in animal products (beef, eggs, chicken, and fish). Choline can be found in plants, but in much smaller amounts (soy, beans, Brussels sprouts, broccoli, and cauliflower).

- Nrf2 activators enhance antioxidants and squelch free radicals, protecting our DNA. Curcumin (from turmeric spice), resveratrol (from grape and berry skin), quercetin (from onions), sulforaphane (from broccoli), and catechins (from green tea and chocolate) are all Nrf2 activators, protecting our body from free radicals and oxidative damage.

Supplements (always best to discuss first with your provider):

- Phosphatidylcholine is particularly useful for individuals living a strict vegetarian or vegan lifestyle.

- Digestive enzymes (with ox bile or HCL when necessary) with meals as needed

- Various nutrients activate NRF2 by different mechanisms. So, when taken together (e.g., curcumin with sulforaphane and resveratrol), they work synergistically together, resulting in a more effective response than when they are taken individually.

Lifestyle:

Avoid Inhibitors of Phase 2.5 detoxification:

- Inflammation (commonly caused by gut dysfunction—dysbiosis and leaky gut)

- Oxidative stress (commonly caused by chronic infection, existing disease, sedentary lifestyle, and bad habits)

- Toxins (found in pesticides, pollution, tobacco, alcohol, poor diet, and medications)

Ways to induce Phase 2.5 detoxification:

- Restore gut health (reducing gut inflammation enhances your detoxification pathways).

- Replace deficiencies (stomach acid, digestive enzymes, bile, or flora).

- Remove irritants (food intolerances, bacterial, yeast, or parasitic overgrowth).

- Stay active—movement is medicine! Regular exercise supports stress reduction, digestive function and your sleep cycle. It also actives our Nrf2 pathways, our body's natural mechanism for creating antioxidants and prevent the damage done by free radicals.

- Intermittent fasting (work up to 14-16 hour fasting window). This upregulates our Nrf2 pathways promoting detoxification and induces ATP Binding Cassettes, enhancing the function of transport proteins and cellular detoxification.

Supporting Your Phase 3 Estrogen Detoxification

Since Phase 3 detoxification takes place outside the liver in the microbiome, I will address it in the next chapter.

Chapter 10

Maximize Your Microbiome

Ten Ways to "Maximize Your Microbiome," the Home of Phase 3 Estrogen Detoxification

1. **Move away from the Western-style diet, also known as the Standard American Diet (SAD).** The SAD is high in sugar, refined carbohydrates, saturated fats and meat and low in fiber. This inhibits gut microbial diversity and contributes to poor overall health. On the flip side, the gut microbiome is responsive and resilient. Studies have shown that making a big dietary shift (for example, moving to a plant-based versus an animal-based diet) can change the levels of our gut bacteria and the kinds of genes they express in as little as three to four days.[87]

2. **Incorporate intermittent fasting into your daily lifestyle.** There are many benefits to intermittent fasting. When it comes to gut health specifically, intermittent fasting supports your gut microbiome diversity and function by activating the migrating motor complex (MMC) to enhance gut motility. A healthy MMC dramatically reduces your risk of impaired gut permeability (or leaky gut) and systemic inflammation associated with it.

3. **Eat clean (organic as much as possible) and go green (environmentally safe products).** Environmental chemicals, such as pesticides (glyphosate) found in our food and water,

endocrine disrupting chemicals (BPAs in plastic), air pollution, and heavy metals (arsenic, lead, mercury, and cadmium) all inhibit the function and diversity of the gut microbiome. Becoming more aware and decreasing our exposure to potential toxins in air, food, water, and personal-care and cleaning products are the first steps to restoring a healthy microbiome. The next step is to increase and diversify our daily intake of plant-based foods (fruits, vegetables, beans, and legumes) to enhance the diversity and health of our microbiome.

4. **Critically evaluate the need and use of medications.** Many prescriptions and OTCs (antibiotics, PPIs, and NSAIDs are the most detrimental) distort the integrity of our microbiome. In some situations, medication may indeed be the best choice; yet in far too many situations, medications are quickly prescribed to treat symptoms and do not address the underlying cause of *why* the symptoms are presenting.

5. **Identify and address your chronic stressors.** The elevated cortisol levels associated with chronic stress negatively affect the composition of the gut microbiota and increase gastrointestinal permeability. Ameliorating stress by incorporating a few very basic and simple stress reduction techniques into your day— such as exercise, mediation, sleep, yoga, and deep-breathing exercises—is a great way to maximize the health of your microbiome and improve your overall health and well-being.

6. **Make your sleep routine a priority.** Sleep dysregulation and deprivation alter the composition of the gut microbiome and metabolism. The gut-brain axis is like a two-way street. Yes—sleep dysregulation disrupts the microbiome, and at the same time, inflammation and a disrupted gut microbiome are linked to sleep loss, circadian rhythm misalignment, mood disorders, and metabolic diseases.[88] If you are experiencing

sleep challenges, having difficulty falling or staying asleep, tune into your gut health. A healthy microbiome produces serotonin, which not only impacts our mood, but also converts to melatonin and impacts our sleep. A healthier microbiome can lead to better quality sleep, and the better quality your sleep, the healthier your microbiome.

7. **Moving your body, as movement is medicine.** Our gut microbiome is positively impacted by exercise. One interesting study done in 2017 looked at the differences in the gut microbiota profile between perimenopausal women with an active lifestyle compared to those with a sedentary lifestyle. The results revealed that women who consistently engaged in an active lifestyle, defined as consistent exercise at least at the minimum level recommended by the WHO (three times a week, thirty-minute sessions, at moderate intensity) had an increased abundance of health-promoting bacteria in their microbiota compared to those women with a sedentary lifestyle.[89]

8. **Identifying your food intolerances and sensitivities.** Eating the right food for you makes all the difference, and that's why sometimes eliminating processed foods and eating all organic may not be enough. Food sensitivities are on the rise, affecting up to one-fifth of the world's population, and can lead to severe gut inflammation and barrier dysfunction (leaky gut) and hinder the health and function of your gut microbiome.[90] Identifying your food sensitivities allows you to personalize your diet to maximize your gut heath. A simple blood test (not a skin test, as that tests for allergies not sensitivities) to evaluate for your specific food sensitivities can dramatically improve gut health and your overall quality of your life.

9. **Addressing and correcting your digestive impairments.**
   Sometimes it's best to let your stool do the talking. A
   comprehensive digestive stool analysis test can provide you
   with insightful information, such as the levels of healthy and
   unhealthy gut flora, pathogenic microbes (parasites, yeast,
   and bacteria), levels of digestive enzyme, inflammation,
   and immune function; detect malabsorption of proteins,
   carbohydrates, and fats; and detect levels of short chain
   fatty acid production (a byproduct from the fermentation of
   indigestible fiber by your gut flora). Remember, identifying
   and treating the underlying cause of your symptoms—not just
   treating the symptoms—is always the goal. Stool testing can
   aid in identifying the underlying cause.

10. **Supplementing with key nutrients when needed.** Supplements
    can offer additional benefits when used appropriately (see
    Appendix B for more information on supplementation). I
    encourage you to work with your provider when choosing
    supplements, as quality matters. Some of the more common
    digestive supplements I recommend in my practice include
    bitters or betaine HCL before meals for hypochlorhydria
    (not enough stomach acid); digestive enzymes with meals for
    malabsorption; bile or bile salts for fat absorption (particularly
    for those with gallbladder challenges); pre- and probiotics to
    restore altered gut flora; L-glutamine to reduce inflammation
    and, as research shows, restore intestinal integrity; demulcent
    herbs (aloe vera, slippery elm, deglycyrrhizinated licorice, and
    marshmallow) to coat, sooth, and heal inflamed or irritated
    tissues; and, of course, fiber because fiber is what feeds your
    gut flora, and our major goal is to have a diverse and healthy
    gut microbiome to maximize detoxification, hormone balance,
    and overall health.

Additional Recommendations for Gut Health

As I have mentioned many times throughout this book, the health of your gut directly impacts the health of your hormones. Constipation and gut inflammation, whether induced by diet, lifestyle, stress, medications, or toxins, will contribute to hormone imbalance. To support you on your quest for hormone balance and overall gut health, I want to include a few additional suggestions for you.

What I am referring to here is the use of castor oil packs, coffee enemas, and, when indicated, colonic therapy. At naturopathic medical school, I was trained on the medicinal uses of these therapies. I routinely discuss and often recommend these therapies for my patients, depending upon their specific health status.

Castor Oil Packs

This simple home remedy can have profound effects on your digestive tract. It is by no means a new form of therapy—the medicinal use of castor oil has been around for millennia, dating back to ancient Egyptian times. And still it is overlooked as a treatment in today's medical arena, even in the naturopathic realm.

Castor oil is derived from the plant *Ricinus communis* (castor bean). When it is ingested orally, which is far less common today, it acts as stimulating laxative. However, when applied topically, in the form of a castor oil pack, it provides anti-inflammatory, detoxifying, and immunomodulating effects, and has been shown to be beneficial in alleviating many gastrointestinal symptoms (gas and bloating, constipation, distension, and fullness sensation).[91]

A castor oil pack is simply a piece of flannel cloth that is saturated with castor oil, applied directly to the skin and left in place for up to two hours (*see How to Do a Castor Oil Pack Below*). Typically, the pack is placed over the liver (located on the right upper side of your abdomen just beneath your lower ribs) to stimulate the liver detoxification. It can be placed over your abdomen (over your small and large intestine) to alleviate constipation and other digestive complaints. And it can even be placed over the lower abdomen, the location of your uterus and ovaries, for complaints of uterine fibroids, ovarian cysts, and PMS cramping.

For best results, the castor oil pack needs to be snuggly applied to the skin. The compression of the castor oil pack against the skin is an important component of the treatment, and for that reason, simply rubbing castor oil on the skin does not provide the same benefit. For additional comfort, heat, in the form of a heating pad or hot water bottle, is often added, yet it is not necessary for the treatment to be effective.

The medicinal benefits of castor oil packs are many. They activate the parasympathetic nervous system, thus enhancing peristaltic motility. They stimulate lymphatic circulation, thus reducing edema and swelling. And they facilitate both liver detoxification and bowel elimination. Together, these benefits ultimately aid in supporting hormone balance.

Like any home treatment modality, there are a few minor drawbacks to castor oil pack treatments. One is the time commitment, as each session does require about an hour. Another is that the castor oil itself is a bit sticky, requiring special cleanup. The oil can stain clothing and bedding. As I share with my patients, these are small prices to pay for the benefits they receive.

A few words of caution here: castor oil packs are contraindicated during pregnancy, while breastfeeding, and during menstrual flow.

How to Do a Castor Oil Pack

This is the version as I learned it in medical school, which is slightly modified from the one described in Harvey Grady's article:[92]

Materials Necessary:

- Castor oil (cold pressed is preferred)

- Flannel cloth (wool is preferred over cotton, unless allergic or unavailable)

- Saran/plastic wrap

- Electric heating pad or hot water bottle (optional)

- Towels (darker color is preferred as castor oil will stain)

- Old clothing and bedding (again, castor oil will stain)

- Storage container

Instructions:

1. Fold flannel cloth twice (four layers) into a size large enough to cover the area being treated.

2. Form a slightly larger sized saran/plastic wrap layer.

3. Place folded flannel cloth on top of the saran wrap. Saturate well with castor oil (not dripping).

4. Place saturated cloth directly on your skin over area of treatment with plastic layer on top.

5. Cover with towel and, if available, apply heating pad (low-medium heat) or a hot water bottle.

6. Leave in place for 45–60 minutes with added heat or 90–120 minutes without added heat. *Note: do not use heat if an inner abscess, appendicitis, or diverticulitis is suspected.*

Cleanup:

1. Clean skin with a baking-soda-and-water solution (2 tablespoons of baking soda and 1 quart of water).

2. Flannel cloth may be reused four to six times. Place in storage container in refrigerator between uses.

3. When the flannel cloth is soiled, dispose of it. *DO NOT* wash in washing machine.

4. CAUTION: castor oil will stain clothing and bedding.

Frequency:

One to two times a week as needed is generally safe. Consult your provider regarding your situation.

Coffee Enemas

Enemas are an ancient remedy used to cleanse the lower bowel, which consists of the rectum and sigmoid colon, and prevent what is known as *autotoxification*. The belief was (and, in naturopathic medicine, still is) that when the bowels are not emptying well (e.g., constipation or impaired elimination), toxins within the bowel are reabsorbed and recycled, leading to illness and disease. The enema procedure itself consists of infusing lukewarm-to-room-temperature water, or another liquid, through the anus into the rectum and sigmoid colon. The purpose is to facilitate the elimination of stool and toxins during the bowel evacuation.

The coffee enema was popularized in the 1930s by Dr. Max Gerson during his work in cancer therapies and is still used today for detoxification purposes.[93] According to Gerson's work, coffee enemas cause dilation of the bile ducts, facilitate the excretion of toxic byproducts in the bowel, enhance the glutathione pathway in Phase 2 liver detoxification, and provide a form of dialysis of blood, removing toxic products from across the colonic wall.

Coffee enemas are generally safe when administered appropriately. They are effective, are inexpensive, and can be done in the convenience of your own home. It is important to note that coffee enemas may be contraindicated for:

- Those diagnosed with any rectal or colon disease (Crohn's, ulcerative colitis, or GI bleeding)

- Those with any underlying cardiac, kidney, or lung disease

- Those who are pregnant

It is always best to be evaluated by your provider before initiating coffee enema therapy. For those of you concerned about the potential stimulating effects of the caffeine, using a more diluted coffee solution is always an option. However, research shows the absorption of caffeine differs depending upon the route of delivery. When the caffeine content of both a coffee solution prepared for the coffee enema and a ready-to-drink coffee beverage were equal, the amount of caffeine absorbed during an enema was 3.5 times less than the amount of caffeine absorbed from drinking a cup of coffee.[94]

How to Do a Coffee Enema

There are many different versions of how to prepare and administer a coffee enema at home. Some are much more elaborate that others, recommending the use of stainless steel enema buckets and sieves, or including music and essential oil for relaxation, for example. Although these items may be useful, they are not necessary. My goal is to keep it simple and as convenient as possible to enhance compliance. One simple example of preparing and administering a coffee enema is available at ineedcoffee.com. I share this version with you, as it closely resembles one I learned in medical school and still suggest to my patients. Now, I offer it to you.

Materials Necessary:

1. Reusable enema kit

2. Lubricant (olive oil, coconut oil, or vitamin E)

3. Organic coffee (light to medium roast)

4. Filtered water

5. French press coffee pot (you can also substitute a drip coffee maker with nonbleached filters)

Preparation:

1. Bring four cups of filtered water to a boil.

2. Grind and add four heaping teaspoons of organic coffee to the French press.

3. Pour boiling water over fresh coffee grounds and seep until lukewarm or room temperature, generally about an hour.

4. Press coffee grounds to the bottom of the press.

5. Pour coffee through a nonbleached filter into the enema bag, filtering out any remaining coffee grounds.

Instructions:

Be sure to review and follow the instructions provided within your enema kit before starting. Many people choose to do their coffee enemas in the bathtub, which offers a convenient way to hang the enema bag from the showerhead, as well as being in close proximity to the toilet. If you choose to perform your enema elsewhere—bed, couch, or floor—just be sure to place a protective layer beneath you, as leaking may occur during the procedure. Lubricate the tip of your enema tubing for ease of insertion. Positioning is important. Lying on your left side, with your knees bent up toward your chest, is most often recommended. For some, the buttocks-up position (while on all fours, lower chest forward until you are resting your forehead on your hands) is most comfortable. For others, lying on their back with their feet up works best.

Once in position, insert the enema tubing into your rectum and slowly infuse the coffee enema. The goal is to retain the contents of the enema for up to fifteen minutes, if possible, before evacuating your bowels. Holding in the contents of the coffee enema will feel uncomfortable. Changing position, rolling from your right side to your back, to your left side, and gently massaging your abdomen can support the process. Once you have a strong urge to evacuate your bowels, go ahead and do so. Upon completion, hydration is important to replenish fluids and electrolytes lost during the enema procedure. Drinking plenty of diluted juices or filtered water with added electrolytes helps to rehydrate your body.

How About Colonics?

Even though they are not a do-it-yourself therapy, I wanted to add a few words regarding the use of colonics. Colon hydrotherapy, commonly referred to as *colonics*, offers another treatment option to support overall digestive health and detoxification. Similar to enemas, colonics promote the dilation of bile ducts, enhance bile flow, stimulate intestinal peristalsis, facilitate elimination, and help relieve constipation.

Unlike enemas, colonics are performed in a clinical setting, using specialized medical equipment, and they are administered by trained and certified colon hydrotherapists. The purpose of a colonic is to infuse water through a series of fills and releases throughout the entire colon, not simply the rectum and sigmoid colon as with an enema.

With each fill, the water temperature and pressure are closely monitored by the colon hydrotherapist. With each release, the contents traveling through the clear tubing can be visually evaluated (you do not have to be the one looking) for fecal material, color, consistency, mucus, food particles, and other items, all of which can provide valuable information regarding the health of your gut, a major detoxification organ for your body.

Despite the conventional medical community's ongoing skeptical view of colonic therapy, essentially declaring them useless and potentially dangerous, alternative medicine proponents support colonic therapy and utilize it as an adjunct to a detoxification plan. The use of colon therapy dates back to the ancient Egyptians and the Greeks. There are ancient documents supporting their therapeutic use of colon irrigation by using hollow reeds and gourds to introduce water through the rectum.

As with any procedure, there are some contraindications for colonic therapy. Individuals experiencing any of the following GI conditions may not be a candidate for colonic therapy:

- Bowel resection (colectomy)
- Rectal prolapse
- Polyps or tumors
- Severe hemorrhoids

- Active colon cancers
- Crohn's disease
- Ulcerative colitis
- Diverticulitis
- GI or rectal bleeding

Caution applies to conditions outside of the gastrointestinal tract as well. These include some cardiac conditions, such as hypertension or dysrhythmias; kidney disease; lung disease; and pregnancy. Getting the clearance from your doctor prior to starting colonics is important and is often a requirement by the colon hydrotherapist.

My Personal Experience With Colonics

As part of my ND training, I, along with my fellow medical students, was required to undergo a series of three colonic sessions. I will admit, my first reaction was: *What?! No Way! Why do I have to do that?* Only after the fact did I realize how beneficial this was for me.

Beyond the physical benefits of the colonics, completing the sessions allowed me to experience the process from a patient's perspective. In turn, this allowed me to share my personal account with my patients, helping alleviate their fears and concerns about having colonics. Some of the most common questions I am asked by my patients include:

Will I have an "accident" while lying on the table? This was my first thought and greatest fear as well. The answer is no, there were no accidents. Once the colonic speculum is placed by the colon hydrotherapist and you are positioned on your back, you're ready to go. Anything released travels out through the speculum into the tubing, so there is no leakage.

I am afraid it is going to be painful. Is it? The truth is that a colonic may feel uncomfortable but should not be painful. The more relaxed you are, the less discomfort you will likely feel. You may experience some sensations of pressure and cramping as the water is infused, similar to the sensations experienced with having diarrhea. The first colonic is often the most challenging simply because you do not know exactly what to expect. Being relaxed is helpful, and therefore, subsequent colonics tend to go more smoothly since you know what expect.

How do I prepare for my colonic? I recommend to my patients to hydrate well leading up to and following their colonic. Hydration helps ward off some of the mild fatigue sometimes experienced following a colonic. Eating very lightly the day of the colonic works best for most of my patients.

Will I feel sick after my colonic? A majority of people feel good after having a colonic. In some cases, you may feel a bit more fatigued and sluggish following a colonic, particularly after your first one. It has to do with lingering toxins liberated during your procedure. Your hydration status can significantly reduce these symptoms. I recommend replenishing with electrolytes, not only water, following your colonic. I also recommend replenishing with a balanced probiotic, too.

How often do I need to do colonics? As a starting point for a detoxification plan, I recommend my patients have a series of three colonics. It may take two to three colonics before your body begins to release toxic bile, so treatments are individualized. Depending on your situation, follow the prescription from your provider regarding the number and frequency of colonics.

In summary, I am a proponent of colonic hydrotherapy, but it is not one of the first recommendations I make to my patients, even though it can be a useful adjunct to their detoxification plan. I have learned that moving in a stepwise approach with my patients, one in which they are able to maintain a sense of feeling in control, has proven to be most successful. Jumping into recommending colon hydrotherapy is too overwhelming for many people—it was for me! Instead I choose to start with nutrition and lifestyle approaches (we can all make changes in these areas); then lean into home therapies, such as hydrotherapy, castor oil packs, and coffee enemas; and then, if indicated, I move into prescriptions for colon hydrotherapy.

Key points when considering colonic therapy:

1. You'll need a rectal exam and be cleared by your doctor before starting treatments.

2. Verify the training and certification of your colon hydrotherapist.

3. Hydrate well before and after colonic sessions. (Electrolytes are most helpful after sessions.)

4. Eat lightly on the day of your colonic.

5. Balanced probiotics are recommended following colonics.

6. Mild abdominal cramping may occur during a colonic.

7. The first one is the hardest one. Your job is to breathe and relax to maximize the effects.

8. It may take two to three colonic sessions to get your toxic bile moving.

9. Follow your provider's prescription for frequency.

Chapter 11

Moving Forward With Daily Detox Practices

Moving Forward With Daily Detox Practices

As I mentioned in the introduction, my intention in writing this book is to deliberately share critically important health information with the world, as it is my mission to move the world toward wellness. Women come into my practice every day suffering needlessly, desperately seeking support and answers for their hormone health challenges. For years, I have shared with my patients exactly what I have finally put into this book.

This book fully exposes the truth behind the worldwide silent epidemic of estrogen dominance: what it is, why it's concerning, how it's occurring, and its negative health consequences. This book also provides you with the solution to preventing, treating, and reversing estrogen dominance and restoring overall health. The solution lies within each of us, whether we have genetic SNPs or not.

The solution is maximizing your gut health. Who knew that the health of our gut determined the health of our hormones? Now you do. You know the role your lymphatics, gallbladder, bile, liver, and microbiome play in regulating hormones. The information you now have at your fingertips by no means provides you with a quick-fix solution. It is a lifestyle plan and a lifetime tool you can use to restore and maintain your hormones and improve your overall health.

Okay. I admit, there is a large volume of information within this book and for some of you this information can seem overwhelming. To some, it may seem like learning an entirely new language. To others who may be more familiar with naturopathic approaches to health, it may open up additional options for you. In either case, you may be asking yourself, where do I start?

Don't overthink it. Start from right where you are.

For some, it may start with diet changes—moving away from processed food to organic foods. For others, it may be a lifestyle change—establishing a set sleep/wake schedule. And for others, it may be cleaning up their environment—throwing out toxic beauty and cleaning supplies and replacing them with healthier items. Keep in mind this is a process, and like any process, it is not intended to be done all at once.

Your prior knowledge and experience along with your current level of health may dictate how aggressively you choose to act. For many of you, I hope this information entices you to seek a licensed naturopathic doctor to work with through your process. (See naturopathic.org to find a listing). In any case, let's look at the next steps you can take.

Steps to Maximizing Your Gut to Harmonize Your Hormones

The following five steps are an abbreviated version of the process I use with my patients in clinical practice. These five steps will guide you on your natural path to hormone health. They are straightforward and relatively easy to implement. For those of you desiring more support with the process or who wish to delve deeper, please visit drjunestevens.com.

1. **Look:** What do you see when you slow down enough to focus on yourself and your surroundings—your diet, your lifestyle, your habits, your home/office surroundings, your sleep, your

stressors? Is there room for improvement in these areas? If so, do not just think about them, write them down. This helps you get organized and move forward with developing your plan.

2. **Listen**: What is your body attempting to tell you? Symptoms are your body's way of asking for help. Honor them. Are you experiencing fluid retention and bloating? Maybe your lymph flow is sluggish. Do you feel fullness, nausea, and discomfort after eating fatty foods? Maybe your bile is too thick and sticky. Are you feeling fatigued, irritable, headachy, and constipated? Maybe your liver is congested. Are you struggling with irritable bowels, sleep challenges, and weight gain? Maybe your microbiome is out of balance. Make a complete list of all your unwanted symptoms; then go back and review the sections of this book that apply most to you and your situation.

3. **Remove**: This is where you let go and get rid of the things you discovered are not serving you on your quest for hormone balance and better health. Decreasing your body's exposure and lowering your body's toxic burden are the goals in the removal process. Please remember, this is a process (a lifestyle change is not a quick fix) and is best done in stages, not all at once. For additional support, revisit the removal process outlined in Chapter 6 to guide you along this path.

4. **Replace**: Removing things from our lives is easier and much more successful when you have something else to replace those items with. Even small changes can have a significant impact. Over time, our healthier daily choices and habits synergistically support our body's natural detoxification pathways, enhancing their function and efficiency. Revisit the replacement process outlined in Chapter 6 to guide you along this path.

5. **Follow**. Staying on course can be challenging at times. We all know stress is part of life and life gets busy. We also know that unexpected things and unforeseen events happen (COVID-19 is a great example) that can derail us from our path. The thing to remember in all life situations is the fact that we have the ability to make choices, and the consistency of our choices is what matters in the long haul. If you find you are off your path, no problem—stop and repeat steps 1 to 4 to get back on. If you find you need help, seek assistance. To assist with staying on course, I share with you what I refer to as *Daily Detox Practices*.

Daily Detox Practices to Maintain Gut and Hormone Balance

1. Consume only clean food, water, and air.

2. Avoid toxic people, places, thoughts, and things.

3. Move your body and your bowels every day.

4. Incorporate hydrotherapy into your hygiene routine.

5. Sweat every day through exercise, or a hot Epsom salt bath, or Far Infrared Sauna.

6. Nourish yourself with nature.

7. Focus on sleep and maintain a set sleep/wake cycle.

8. Practice gratitude daily.

Parting Words

Now that you have learned this information and have many resources available to you, your next step is to take action.

How are you going to use this information for your own health?

How are you going to modify your diet, lifestyle, and environment to maximize your gut health and hormone balance?

Are you going to share this information with others?

Many women (and men too) are struggling with hormone imbalance and gut issues, and they could greatly benefit from the knowledge you have learned from this book. I love practicing as a naturopathic doctor, and sharing my knowledge with others is one of the most rewarding parts of what I do, yet it means absolutely nothing unless it gets implemented and results in positive outcomes for others.

First and foremost, I ask that you use this information for yourself to restore and maintain your own gut and hormone health. Additionally, I ask you to please pass this information along to anyone who may be interested. I firmly believe that by helping others reach their greatest health potential, together, we can all move the world toward wellness.

Appendix A

Laboratory Testing—A Conventional and Functional Testing Reference Guide

Lymphatics Testing

Unfortunately, lymphatic testing is challenging. There really are no conventional or functional laboratory tests available at this time to determine the actual status of your lymphatic flow, nor are there tests available to determine how your lymphatic system may be impacting your overall hormonal balance. Therefore, the most accurate ways to determine if lymphatic congestion is likely present and how it may be impacting your hormone balance is by tuning in to your body's signs and symptoms and evaluating your diet and lifestyle.

Gallbladder/Bile Testing

Conventional Blood Tests:

- **Complete Blood Count (CBC)**. This test may show an elevated white blood cell (WBC) count in the case of gallbladder infection.

- **Liver Enzymes** (*alanine aminotransferase* (ALT), *aspartate aminotransferase* (AST), *gamma-glutamyl transferase* (GGT). These may be elevated in the case of biliary obstruction.

- **Bilirubin**. May be elevated as a result of limited excretion secondary to gallstones.

Conventional Diagnostic Imaging Tests:

- **Abdominal ultrasound.** Most commonly used imaging test to determine size of gallstones, yet provides no information on inflammation.

- **Abdominal X-rays.** May detect some calcium-containing gallstones, yet not all types.

- **Computed tomography (CT).** Useful for detecting an infected or ruptured gallbladder but may not detect stones.

- **Magnetic resonance imaging (MRI).** May detect stones within the bile ducts but may not detect infections.

- **Endoscopic retrograde cholangiopancreatography (ERCP).** Considered the gold standard test to diagnose and remove stones blocking bile ducts, yet complications can arise in up to 10 percent of those treated.

- **Hepatobiliary iminodiacetic acid (HIDA) scan.** A test to evaluate for acute gallbladder inflammation and bile duct obstruction and to measure how efficient your gallbladder is at releasing bile, otherwise known as gallbladder ejection fraction.

Liver Testing

Conventional blood tests (The following blood tests are often evaluated as a group, rather than isolated tests, to determine liver health):

- **Liver enzymes (*alanine aminotransferase* (ALT), *aspartate aminotransferase* (AST), *gamma-glutamyl transferase* (GGT)).** Elevated in cases of biliary obstruction or liver cell injury.

- **Bilirubin**. A waste product processed through the liver. Elevated levels may indicate impaired liver function.

- *Alkaline phosphatase* (**ALP**). May be elevated with liver inflammation or injury and bile duct blockage.

- **Albumin**. The main protein produced in the liver. Low levels may indicate impaired liver function.

- *Lactate dehydrogenase* (**LD**). May be elevated in cases of liver damage or injury, yet can be elevated in many other disorders.

- *Prothrombin time* (**PT**). The time it takes your blood to clot; thus, an increased PT may indicate liver damage.

Conventional Diagnostic Imaging Tests (most useful in detecting liver structure or damage, yet less useful for evaluating liver function or detoxification):

- **Abdominal X-rays**. Able to detect abdominal calcifications, masses, perforations, or obstructions.

- **Abdominal ultrasound**. Useful in determining the size and location of organs, and helpful in detecting cysts, tumors, abscesses, fluid accumulation, obstructions, and aneurysms.

- **Computed tomography (CT)**. Indicated to evaluate unexplained abdominal pain particularly when other testing is inconclusive. CT can detect injury, bleeding, infections, tumors, fluid accumulation, abscesses, and obstructions. CT is considered the most sensitive imaging test for the evaluation of liver metastasis.

- **Magnetic resonance imaging (MRI)**. Can detect liver conditions such as hepatitis and hemochromatosis and may be the most sensitive imaging test for steatosis, or fatty liver disease.

Specialty Lab Testing (Functional Medicine Testing)

When it comes to evaluating the health and function of your gut and your hormones, conventional standardized testing, although useful, most often is simply not enough. Tests, such as an endoscopy or colonoscopy, are helpful in determining tissue injury such as gastritis, esophagitis, or ulcers, as well as structural changes—such as hiatal hernias, polyps, and diverticulosis—yet these tests are not useful in determining the function of your gut.

Specialty testing, often referred to as *functional medicine testing*, provides a better solution. Functional medicine testing provides a deeper look into how your body is functioning:

- Is your body metabolizing and excreting your hormones efficiently?

- Is your body absorbing nutrients from your diet?

- Are you suffering from food intolerances and, unknowingly, eating the wrong foods?

- Are you unknowingly carrying around high levels of toxicants (pesticides, heavy metals, or xenoestrogens) in your body?

Functional medicine testing provides the answers to such questions and thus aids in determining the root cause of your symptoms or condition, allowing for personalized treatments.

A number of laboratory companies now offer specialty testing, and this number is growing rapidly. Both the wellness industry and consumer demand are the driving forces behind this growth. Many companies now offer testing kits directly to you, the consumer, while others require you to go through your provider for testing.

I compiled the following list of companies offering different types of specialty testing based on my years of personal experience utilizing them in clinical practice with great success. I am now sharing this information with you, and I encourage you to also share this list with your providers. This information is vital and needs to be shared. Please be advised, not all medical providers will be familiar with functional medicine testing, nor will they be open to it. You may want to consider finding a naturopathic doctor (see naturopathic.org to find a listing) or a functional medicine or integrative practitioner in your area to assist you.

Specialty Testing: Sex Hormones (Estrogens, Progesterone, and Testosterone)					
Lab Company	**Name**	**Tests for**	**Sample**	**Contact**	**Notes**
Precision Analytical	DUTCH Complete Test	Sex hormones Metabolites	Dried urine	dutchtest. com	*Tests to determine how efficiently your body metabolizes hormones.*
Precision Analytical	DUTCH Cycle Mapping	Monthly pattern of estrogen and progesterone metabolites	Dried urine	dutchtest. com	
ZRT Laboratories	Hormone Trio or Female Profile	Sex hormones Metabolites	Saliva, Blood spot, Dried urine	zrtlab.com	
Diagnos-Techs	Post or Peri-Menopause Panel Cycling Female Panel	Sex hormones	Saliva	diagnostechs. com	

Specialty Testing: Adrenal Hormones (Cortisol, DHEA)					
Lab Company	**Name**	**Tests for**	**Sample**	**Contact**	**Notes**
Precision Analytical	DUTCH Adrenal	Adrenal hormones Metabolites	Saliva Urine	dutchtest.com	
Diagnos-Techs	Adrenal Stress Index (ASI)	Adrenal hormones	Saliva	diagnostechs.com	
ZRT Laboratory	Adrenal Stress Profile	Adrenal hormones	Saliva	zrtlab.com	

Specialty Testing: Digestive Function					
Lab Company	**Name**	**Tests for**	**Sample**	**Contact**	**Notes**
Great Plains Laboratory	Organic Acids Test (OAT)	Fungal and Bacterial metabolites	Urine	greatplainslaboratory.com	
Genova Diagnostics	GI Effects	Absorption Inflammation Immunology Microbiome	Stool	gdx.net	
Doctor Data, Inc.	CDSA with Parasitology	Absorption Inflammation Immunology Beneficial flora Dysbiotic flora Yeast Parasites Pathogens	Stool	doctorsdata.com	
Diagnostic Solutions Laboratory	GI Map	Absorption Inflammation Immunology Beneficial flora Dysbiotic flora Yeast Parasites Pathogens	Stool	diagnosticsolutionslab.com	

Specialty Testing: Microbiome Testing					
Lab Company	**Name**	**Tests for**	**Sample**	**Contact**	**Notes**
Doctors Data, Inc.	GI–360	Microbiome abundance and diversity	Stool	doctorsdata.com	
Diagnostic Solutions Laboratory	GI-MAP	Microbiome abundance and diversity	Stool	diagnosticsolutionslab.com	
Genova Diagnostics	GI Effects	Microbial abundance and diversity	Stool	gdx.net	

Specialty Testing: Impaired Intestinal Permeability (Leaky Gut)					
Lab Company	**Name**	**Tests for**	**Sample**	**Contact**	**Notes**
Cyrex Laboratory	The Array 2	LPS Occludin Zonulin Actomysin Protein Antibody	Blood	cyrexlabs.com	
Doctors Data, Inc.	Zonulin	Zonulin	Blood, Stool	doctorsdata.com	
Diagnostic Solutions Laboratory	Zonulin	Zonulin	Stool	diagnosticsolutionslab.com	
Genova Diagnostic	Zonulin Family Peptides	Zonulin Family Peptides	Stool	gdx.net	
Genova Diagnostics	Intestinal Permeability Assessment	Lactulose/ Mannitol Test	Urine	gdx.net	
Doctors Data, Inc.	Intestinal Permeability	Lactulose/ Mannitol Test	Urine	doctorsdata.com	

Specialty Testing: Irritable Bowel Syndrome (IBS)					
Lab Company	**Name**	**Tests for**	**Sample**	**Contact**	**Notes**
Gemelli Biotech	IBS-Smart	Levels of anti-CdtB and anti-vinculin antibodies	Blood	ibssmart. com	*The first test available to diagnose IBS.*

Specialty Testing: Small Intestinal Bacterial Overgrowth (SIBO)/ Intestinal Methanogen Overgrowth (IMO)					
Lab Company	**Name**	**Tests for**	**Sample**	**Contact**	**Notes**
Genova Diagnostics	SIBO Test	Methane and Hydrogen levels	Breath test	gdx.net	*I recommend the three-hour sample collection.*
The SIBO Test	SIBO Test	Methane and hydrogen levels	Breath test	sibotest. com	
Gemelli Biotech	Trio-Smart	Methane Hydrogen Hydrogen sulfide	Breath test	triosmart-breath.com	*Groundbreaking new test made available in Oct 2020. The first test available for measuring Hydrogen Sulfide levels.*

Specialty Testing: Beta-glucuronidase					
Lab Company	Name	Tests for	Sample	Contact	Notes
Doctors Data, Inc.	Beta-Glucu-ronidase	Beta-glucuro-nidase levels	Stool	doctorsda-ta.com	
Diagnostics Solutions Laboratory	Beta-Glucu-ronidase	Beta-glucuro-nidase levels	Stool	diagnost-icsolution-slab.com	
Genova Diagnos-tics	Beta-Glucu-ronidase	Beta-glucuro-nidase levels	Stool	gdx.net	

Specialty Testing: Nutritional Status Evaluation					
Lab Company	Name	Tests for	Sample	Contact	Notes
SpectraCell Laborato-ries	Micronutrient Test (MNT)	Tests 31 differ-ent vitamins, minerals, ami-no acids, and antioxidants	Blood	spectracell.com	
Genova Diagnostics Laboratory	NutrEval	Evaluates the body's need for: Antioxidants B-vitamins Key minerals Essential fatty acids Amino acids Digestive, microbiome, mitochondrial and methyla-tion support Toxic exposure	Blood, Urine	gdx.net	

Specialty Testing: IgG Food Sensitivity

Lab Company	Name	Tests for	Sample	Contact	Notes
AlleTess Medical Laboratory	AlleTess (Candida Albicans and H. pylori ADD ON tests available)	Tests for 96–184 foods	Blood or blood spot	foodallergy.com	
KBMO Diagnostics	The FIT Test (Candida Albicans and H. pylori ADD ON tests available)	Tests for 176 foods	Blood or blood spot	kbmodiagnostics.com	*Additional environmental and food allergy panels also available.*
Immuno Laboratories	BloodPrint Test (Candida Albicans and H. pylori ADD ON tests available)	Tests for 88–200 foods	Blood	immunolabs.com	

Specialty Testing: Toxicity Testing

Lab Company	Name	Tests for	Sample	Contact	Notes
Great Plains Laboratory	GLP-TOX Profile	Environmental toxicity panel	Urine	greatplainslaboratory.com	
Great Plains Laboratory	MycoTox Profile	Mold metabolite panel	Urine	greatplainslaboratory.com	
Great Plains Laboratory	Glyphosate	Glyphosate ("Round UP" testing)	Urine	greatplainslaboratory.com	
Great Plains Laboratory	Heavy Metals	Heavy metal testing with or without essential elements	Urine Stool Blood Hair	greatplainslaboratory.com	

Doctors Data Inc.	Heavy Metals	Heavy metals testing with or without essential elements	Urine Stool Blood Hair	doctorsdata.com	
Quicksilver Scientific	Heavy Metals	Heavy metals	Blood Urine	quicksilverscientific.com	*Experts in mercury.*
OligoScan	Heavy Metals	Heavy metals Essential elements Vitamins B6, B12, folate, C, D, E, and A	Dermal scan (in-office testing only)	oligoscan.fr/lg/en/index.html	

Specialty Testing: Detoxification Profiles					
Lab Company	**Name**	**Tests for**	**Sample**	**Contact**	**Notes**
Doctors Data, Inc.	Hepatic Detox Profile	D-glucaric acid (Phase 1 function) Mercapturic acids levels (Phase 2 function)	Urine	www.doctorsdata.com	
Genova Diagnostics	DetoxiGenomic Profile	SNPs evaluation for Phase 1 and Phase 2 detox	Oral swab	gdx.net	*Some individual SNP testing also available (e.g., MTHFR, COMT, GSTM)*
Great Plains Laboratories	Organic Acids Test (OAT)	Yeast/bacterial metabolites Krebs Cycle Glutathione Nutritional markers	Urine	greatplainslaboratory.com	

Specialty Testing: Genetic Testing					
Note: I recommend working with your provider when evaluating any of your genetic results.					
Lab Company	**Name**	**Tests for**	**Sample**	**Contact**	**Notes**
StrateGene	StrateGene Genetic Analysis	Your genetics	Saliva Oral Swab	strategene. me	*Provides full service and the most clinically relevant SNPs information.*
23 and Me	Health and Ancestry	Your genetics	Saliva	23andme. com	*Offer you raw data needing further evaluation for clinically relevant SNP information.*
AncestryD-NA	Ancestry-Health	Your genetics	Saliva	ancestry. com	
Prometh-ease	An online DNA reporting tool that evaluates for your SNPs based upon you uploading your raw genetic data to this site	Does not test your genetics	N/A	prometh-ease.com	*Provides a large volume of information, but doesn't provide information on diet, lifestyle, or environmental factors impacting your SNPs.*

Appendix B

Supplementation Support

Every day, patients ask me questions regarding supplements. Some frequently asked questions are:

- *Is this a good supplement for me to take?*

- *What do you think of the quality of this supplement?*

- *Is it okay to take this supplement along with my prescription medications?*

- *Why is this brand so much more expensive than the others?*

First, I'm glad my patients ask me these questions, and I hope they keep asking them. These are important questions, and the correct answer may vary from person to person.

Despite being seen as a more natural approach to health, supplements can be powerful and, in some cases, potentially dangerous; therefore, they should not be taken lightly. Just because they are touted as natural does not mean they are safe for everyone.

There are many factors to consider, such as:

- Quality
- Potency
- Bioavailability
- How closely they resemble food
- Additives and fillers

Supplements have become a huge part of the health and wellness industry, but please remember that they are intended to supplement a healthy diet and lifestyle, not serve as a replacement for poor diet and lifestyle choices. My motto regarding supplementation has always been and continues to be: *Food first. Then supplements. Then medication.*

Reviewing supplements with patients and providing them with access to obtaining top-quality, physician-line, nutritional supplements is a service I offer to all my patients. The quality of supplements is of the utmost importance, and I am pleased to say there are many very reputable nutraceutical companies who have gone the extra mile, adhering to stringent regulations set by the Food and Drug Administration in order to maintain Good Manufacturing Practices (GMP) to produce their physician-grade products. Unfortunately, there are far too many companies who do not have the interest of the consumer at heart. Just how prevalent is this?

In February 2015, after completing its investigation, the New York Attorney General's office issued cease and desist letters to four major retailers—GNC, Target, Walgreens, and Walmart. The investigation found that most of the store-brand supplements were found to contain contaminants not identified on ingredient labels. Also, only 21 percent of supplement tests had identified DNA from plant species listed on label.[95] Yes—the active ingredients were nonexistent in most of the bottles of supplements. What is even more disturbing was that the level of contaminants was undisclosed on the labels. This poses additional health risks, such as allergic reactions.

A similar episode occurred in February 2019, when the FDA took action against seventeen companies, both foreign and domestic. These companies were illegally selling products on websites and social media, many sold as dietary supplements, when they were actually unapproved new drugs or misbranded drugs. They claimed these supplements prevented, treated, or cured Alzheimer's disease, as well as a number of other serious diseases and health conditions.[96]

I always share this information with my patients, and now I am sharing it with you. My intention is to shed light on just how vulnerable we may be when it comes to purchasing supplements. Once again, quality matters. A large bottle of product at a cheap price found on the internet is likely not the best option. In fact, it may be more harmful than helpful. For best results, work with a provider who will assist you with access to reputable companies and quality products. Your provider will also aid you in choosing the right supplements for you based upon your given situation.

When restoring and maintaining hormone balance, I always focus on my patients' dietary and lifestyle modifications first. In many cases, diet and lifestyle may not be enough. Additional supplementation with key nutrients provides additional benefits. Since each person's individual needs are variable, dosages are also variable. Dosing may depend on your body weight, other existing health conditions, genetics, and the integrity of your gut function. You can take all the supplements in the world, but if you are not able to absorb them well, you are less likely to get the positive outcome you are searching for. As well, if you are not eliminating well, other side effects are likely to manifest.

If you are taking or are planning to take supplements, keep in mind they come in many different forms (capsules, tablets, powders, liquids, tinctures, teas), dosages (milligrams, grams, milliliters, drops), and concentrations. The dosages provided in the following charts are simply a guideline, and I highly recommend you discuss any supplementation with your provider.

Reference Guide for Supplementation – Dr. June's Top 10 Lists

Dr. June's Top 10 for Stress/Anxiety (High Cortisol)

Stress/Anxiety (High Cortisol)	Dosage	Notes
Omega-3 fatty acids (fish oil)	1,000–3,000 mg (daily with food)	Calming to the nervous system and adrenal glands, modulating the stress response
Magnesium	One to two 125 mg capsules (1–4 times a day)	Lowers cortisol and promotes relaxation; chelated forms (bisglycinate, malate, taurate) are best for absorption
B-complex	One capsule (1–2 times a day)	Reduces stress and supports cognition and mood
Vitamin C	500 mg (1–3 times daily)	Restorative to the adrenal glands, reduces stress
Phosphatidylserine (PS)	400–800 mg (daily)	Reduces cortisol and supports mood under stress
L-theanine	100–400 mg (daily)	Reduces cortisol to support cognition and memory
Ashwagandha	300 mg (twice daily)	Adaptogen (Balances stress hormones)
Rhodiola	200 mg (twice daily)	Adaptogen (Reduces anxiety, supports mood)
Cordyceps	400 mg (twice daily)	An adaptogenic medicinal mushroom that balances cortisol and modulates the immune system
Lemon balm	100–300 mg (daily)	Supports calmness, memory, and focus under stress
Dr. June's Top Formulas		
Stress support	One capsule (1–3 times daily with meals)	Learn more at: nutritionalscripts. com/drjunestevens
Adrenal (energy and stress relief)	One to two capsules (1–2 times daily)	Learn more at: nutritionalscripts. com/drjunestevens

Dr. June's Top 10 for Stress/Fatigue (Low Cortisol)

Stress/Fatigue (Low Cortisol)	Dosage	Notes
Omega-3 fatty acids (fish oil)	1,000–3,000 mg (daily with food)	Calming to the nervous system and adrenal glands and modulates the stress response
B-complex	One capsule (1–2 times daily)	Supports energy, cognition, and mood
Vitamin C	500 mg (1–3 times daily)	Restorative to the adrenal glands
Licorice root extract	200 mg (1–2 times daily)	Delays the breakdown of cortisol to sustain energy; best taken in the morning and early afternoon to not disrupt sleep. *CAUTION: This herb can elevate blood pressure*
Ashwagandha	300 mg (twice daily)	Adaptogen (balances stress hormones)
Panax ginseng	200 mg (twice daily)	Reduces fatigue, supports cognition and memory
MACA	1,000–3,000 mg (daily)	Supports energy, mood, sleep, and cognition *CAUTION: This adaptogen may have mild estrogenic effects*
American skullcap	400–1,200 mg (daily)	Can be restorative following long periods of physical and emotional stress
Eleutherococcus	200–400 mg (daily)	Adaptogen (supports energy, metabolism, and immunity)

Adrenal cortex	500 mg (1–3 times daily)	Glandular products (often combined with other nutrients) are used in significantly depleted states They provide a balance of multiple factors to promote the health, growth, and maintenance of organs and glands *CAUTION: Only take glandular products under the supervision of your provider*
Adrenal glandular	250 mg (1–2 times daily)	
Dr. June's Top Formulas		
Burn Out Reliever	One capsule (1–3 times daily)	Learn more at: nutritionalscripts.com/drjunestevens
Adrenal Boost	One tablet (1–2 times daily)	Learn more at: nutritionalscripts.com/drjunestevens

Dr. June's Top 10 for Restorative Sleep

Restorative Sleep	Dosage	Notes
Melatonin	0.5–3 mg tablet (1 hour before bed)	A natural sleep hormone produced from serotonin to induce sleep
5-HTP	100–300 mg capsule (1 hour before bed)	Precursor to melatonin (supports mood, appetite, and sleep)
GABA (gamma aminobutyric acid)	100–300 mg capsule (1–2 times daily)	An inhibitory neurotransmitter that produces calming effects for the brain and nervous system
L Theanine	200–400 mg capsule (1–2 times daily)	Modulates effects on the brain promoting relaxation
Magnesium	125–250 mg capsule (1–2 times daily)	Lowers cortisol and promotes relaxation; maintains the normal circadian rhythms, improving sleep quality
Magnolia bark with phellodendron bark	350–700 mg capsule (at bedtime)	Supports your natural GABA function, calms the brain to promote both falling and staying asleep, and improves REM sleep

Passionflower	200–400 mg capsule (1–2 times daily)	Calming; induces sleep and muscle relaxation; commonly consumed as a tea or in liquid tincture form
Lemon balm	300 mg capsule (1–2 times daily)	A calming and mild sedative effect that supports sleep quality
Lavender oil (Lavela)	80 mg capsule (before bed)	Calming to the nervous system, improving the quality and duration of sleep
Valerian	400 mg capsule (before bed)	Inhibits the breakdown GABA, promoting calmness, relaxation, and a feeling of tranquility
Dr. June's Top Formulas		
Tranquility (herb blend)	1–2 capsules before bed	Learn more at: nutritionalscripts.com/drjunestevens
Cortisol Stabilizer	1–2 capsules before bed	Learn more at: nutritionalscripts.com/drjunestevens

Dr. June's Top 10 for Lymphatics[97]

Lymph Movers (Tincture Form)	Dose	Notes
Poke root	1–10 drops (1–3 times daily)	Useful for swollen lymph nodes, tissues, and skin conditions like boils or eczema. *CAUTION: This is an extremely powerful herb with toxic properties. It should be used under the supervision of your provider.*
Burdock root	20–60 drops (1–4 times daily)	Supportive to the skin, kidneys, liver, gallbladder, and mucus membranes.
Red clover	10–60 drops (1–4 times daily)	Has an affinity for the lungs and neck, useful for coughs, throat congestion, swollen glands, and skin issues.
Cleavers	30–75 drops (1–3 times daily)	Supports the kidneys and bladder, reduces stones and fibrocystic tissue, and useful in skin conditions.

Oregon grape root	10–60 drops (1–4 times daily)	Stimulates sluggish GI tract, respiratory, and urinary tracts; GI infections, liver congestion, gallbladder stasis, and skin conditions (acne, eczema, or psoriasis).
Goldenseal	10–60 drops (1–4 times daily)	Contains the alkaloid berberine, which stimulates gut motility and liver and gallbladder function; increases bile secretion; and provides antimicrobial activity against bacteria, yeast, viruses, and parasites. *CAUTION: May exacerbate low adrenal symptoms.*
Gold thread	10–60 drops (1–4 times daily)	Contains the alkaloid berberine, which stimulates gut motility and liver and gallbladder function, increases bile secretion, and provides antimicrobial activity against bacteria, yeast, viruses, and parasites.
Echinacea	10–75 drops (1–4 times daily)	Has immune-modulating effects protecting the gut from infections, decreasing inflammation, and stimulating gastric healing
Figwort	10–30 drops (1–4 times daily)	Relieves congestion in GI tract, liver, and pelvic region. Useful for enlarged lymph glands, hemorrhoids, and skin conditions.
Wild indigo root	2–10 drops (1–4 times daily)	Actives the immune system and promotes healthy cellular metabolism and waste removal to support healthy tissues. *CAUTION: This herb is toxic in high doses. Use under supervision of your provider.*
Dr. June's Top Formulas		
Lymphagogue Compound	30–60 drops (3–4 times daily)	Learn more at: us.fullscript.com/welcome/drjune
Herbal Detox	1 dropper (2–3 times daily)	Learn more at: us.fullscript.com/welcome/drjune

Dr. June's Top 10 for Bile and Gallbladder

Bile and Gallbladder Support	Dose	Notes
Phosphatidylcholine	350–800 mg (with meals)	A key component of bile. Supports its slippery texture, promoting easier flow and reduced risk for gallstones.
Ox bile	125–250 mg (with meals)	Particularly useful for those without a gallbladder. Emulsifies fats to enhance their absorption and promotes gut health.
Lipase	60–120 mg (with meals)	The primary enzyme for fat absorption
Taurine	250–500 mg (with meals)	Helps increase the natural production of bile acids in the liver
Ginger	250–500 mg (1–2 times daily)	As a bitter, it stimulates bile flow and gastric motility
Turmeric	100–500 mg (1–2 times daily)	As a bitter, it stimulates bile production and flow.
Gentian root	100–200 mg (1–3 times daily)	A strong bitter that stimulates all secretions, gastric motility, and enhances nutrient absorption
Barberry bark	250–500 mg (1–2 times daily)	Stimulates production and flow of bile, enhances liver function and gastric motility
Burdock root	250–500 mg (1–2 times daily)	Stimulates lymph and bile flow, enhances liver and digestive function, acts as a mild laxative, and restores hormone balance
Dandelion root	150–500 mg (1–2 times daily)	Increases bile flow and decreases liver congestion
Dr. June's Top Formulas		
Liver and GB support	1–2 capsules (with meals)	Learn more at: nutritionalscripts.com/drjunestevens
Digestion GB	1–2 capsules (with meals)	Learn more at: us.fullscripts.com/welcome/drjune

Dr. June's Top 10 for Liver Support

Liver Support	Dose	Notes
N-acetyl cysteine (NAC)	600 mg (twice daily)	An amino acid the body uses to produce glutathione
Glutathione (liposomal form)	500 mg (¼–½ tsp under tongue twice daily)	One of our body's most potent natural antioxidants; essential for detoxification
Alpha lipoic acid	250–600 mg (daily)	Protects the liver from oxidative damage
Milk thistle	100–250 mg (1–4 times daily)	Protects liver and kidney cells and activates the regenerative capacity of liver cells
Artichoke leaf	200–500 mg (1–2 times daily)	Protects the liver and supports liver cell regeneration
Dandelion root	350–500 mg (1–2 times daily)	Increases bile flow and decreases liver congestion
Burdock root	250–500 mg (1–2 times daily)	Stimulates lymph and bile flow, enhances liver and digestive function, acts as a mild laxative, and restores hormone balance
Bupleurum root	200 mg (1–2 times daily)	A staple herb in Chinese medicine for detoxification and used in many formulas; a member of the *Apiaceae* family of plants, it's known to support estrogen metabolism
Yellow dock root	350 mg (1–2 times daily)	Naturally rich in iron, reduces liver congestion, supports fat absorption, and stimulates motility
Gentian	100–200 mg (1–3 times daily)	A strong bitter that stimulates all secretions and gastric motility and enhances nutrient absorption
Dr. June's Top Formulas		
Liver and GB support	One to two capsules (2–3 times daily)	Learn more at: nutritionalscripts.com/ drjunestevens
Milk thistle plus	One capsule	Learn more at: nutritionalscripts.com/ drjunestevens

Dr. June's Top 10 for Intestinal Microbiome

Gut and Microbiome Support	Dosage	Notes
Bitters (potency varies)	30–60 drops in water (15 minutes before meals)	Stimulates the flow of stomach acid, bile, and digestive enzymes promoting overall gut function
Prebiotics/probiotics (sources and strains variable)	10–100 billion (1–2 times daily)	Probiotics induce positive changes to the gut microbiome by reducing levels of harmful bacteria and enhancing levels of beneficial flora
Fiber (sources variable)	3–12 grams (in divided doses daily— start with lower dose)	Fiber feeds our flora and promotes a more diverse and abundant microbiome *CAUTION: With some active conditions, e.g., colitis, diverticulitis, Crohn's, obstruction*
Digestive enzymes (some may contain added HCL or and/or ox bile)	1–2 capsules (with meals)	Essential for the breakdown and absorption of food: protease for proteins, amylase for carbohydrates, and lipase for fats; these positively impact the diversity and abundance of the microbiome
Betaine/HCL	300–500 mg (1–2 capsules with meals)	Essential for protein breakdown, provides antimicrobial properties and supports stomach and intestinal pH balance, promoting a healthy microbiome
L–glutamine	3000–5000 mg (2–3 times daily)	Soothing and restorative to gut inflammation (Leaky Gut); increases SIgA levels, enhancing gut immunity; supports a healthy Firmicutes-to-Bacteroidetes ratio in the microbiome
Ginger	250–500 mg (1–3 times daily)	Supports gut motility and enhances short chain fatty acid production by modulating the gut microbiome.
Slippery elm	1500–2000 mg (1–2 times daily between meals)	Increases the abundance of health-promoting gut flora (*Bifidobacterium, Lactobacillus*, and *Bacteroides)* while inhibiting disease-inducing bacteria (*Citrobacter freundii* and *Klebsiella pneumoniae)*

Deglycyrrhizinated licorice (DGL)	300 mg (1–4 times daily, after meals)	Increases the abundance of health-promoting gut flora (*Bifidobacterium*, *Lactobacillus*, and *Bacteroides*) while inhibiting disease-inducing bacteria (*Citrobacter freundii* and *Klebsiella pneumoniae*).
Triphala	500–1000 mg (1–2 times daily)	Increases the abundance of health-promoting gut flora (*Bifidobacterium*, *Lactobacillus*, and *Bacteroides*) while inhibiting disease-inducing bacteria (*Citrobacter freundii* and *Klebsiella pneumoniae*)
Dr. June's Top Formulas		
IBS Powder	One scoop (2–3 times daily)	Learn more at: nutritionalscripts.com/drjunestevens
Fiber Complete	Half to full scoop (1–2 times daily) on an empty stomach)	Learn more at: nutritionalscripts.com/drjunestevens

Dr. June's Top 10 (plus 2) for Estrogen Dominance

Reducing Estrogen Dominance	Dose	Notes
B-vitamins (esp. B2, 3, 6, 12, and folate)	One capsule (1–2 times daily with meals)	Essential for methylation and estrogen detoxification. Supports mood, energy, and sleep.
Magnesium (bisglycinate)	125–250 mg (1–2 times daily)	Essential for COMT enzyme function, estrogen detoxification, and a balanced stress response.

Diindolylmethane (DIM)	100–300 mg (daily)	Potentiates the preferred 2-OH estrogen metabolite pathway of estrogen metabolism.
Calcium D-glucarate	500–1000 mg (twice daily)	Supports Phase 3 estrogen detoxification by lowering Beta-glucuronidase enzyme activity in the microbiome preventing estrogen recycling.
Chrysin	100–200 mg	Decreases aromatase enzyme activity, thus decreasing the conversion of testosterone to estrogen, lowering risk for estrogen dominance.
Milk thistle	100–250 mg (1–4 times daily)	Nutritive, protective, and restorative to liver cells, supports healthy estrogen metabolism.
NAC	600 mg (twice daily)	Enhances Glutathione production necessary for healthy Phase 2 detoxification.
Sulforaphane	100–200 mg (twice daily)	A potent Nrf2 activator that enhances Phase 2 detoxification pathways in the liver and turns on the body's natural production of antioxidants to protect against oxidative stress.
Green tea	100–200 mg (1–2 times daily)	Nrf2 activator supportive to estrogen detoxification by upregulating Phase 2 detoxification and protects against oxidative stress.
Curcumin	100–500 mg (twice daily)	Slows Phase 1 detoxification, decreasing free radical production. At the same time, it enhances Phase 2 detoxification, promoting detoxification.
Resveratrol	100–200 mg (1–2 times daily)	Nrf2 activator supportive to estrogen detoxification by upregulating Phase 2 detoxification and protects against oxidative stress.
Quercetin	100–250 mg (1–2 times daily)	Nrf2 activator supportive to estrogen detoxification by upregulating Phase 2 detoxification and protects against oxidative stress.

Dr. June's Top Formulas		
Estrogen balance	One capsule (1–2 times daily)	Learn more at: nutritionalscripts.com/drjunestevens
B-active plus	One capsule (1–2 times daily)	Learn more at: nutritionalscripts.com/drjunestevens

Other Resources

For those of you feeling inspired and wanting more information, come visit my website at www.drjunestevens.com, where you can join our community and find additional resources. My goal is to share my knowledge and wisdom with you. I ask you to please pass this information along to anyone who may be interested. I firmly believe that by helping others reach their greatest health potential, together, we can all move the world toward wellness.

Books

- *The Complete Guide to Fasting* by Jason Fung, MD (Victory Belt Publishing, 2016)

- *Cooking for Hormone Balance* by Magdalena Wszelaki (HarperOne, 2018)

- *Overcoming Estrogen Dominance* by Magdalena Wszelaki (Hormones & Balance, 2021)

- *Healthy Home Healthy Family* by Nicole Bijlsman, ND (Joshua Books, 2010)

- *Clean, Green & Lean* by Walter Crinnion, ND (Wiley, 2010)

- *The Toxin Solution* by Joseph Pizzorno, ND (HarperOne, 2017)

- *Herbal Medicine* by Sharol Tilgner, ND (Wise Acres, 2009)

- *Dirty Genes* by Ben Lynch, ND (HarperCollins Publishers, 2020)

- *The Hormone Cure* by Sara Gotteried, MD (Scribner, 2013)

- *Creating and Maintaining Balance: A Woman's Guide to Safe, Natural Hormone Health* by Holly Lucille, ND (IMPKT Health, 2004)

- *8 Weeks to Women's Wellness* by Marianne Marchaese, ND (Smart Publications, 2013)

- *Cancer: The Journey From Diagnosis to Empowerment* by Paul Anderson, ND (Lioncrest Publishing, 2020)

- *The Metabolic Approach to Cancer* by Nasha Winters, ND (Chelsea Green Publishing, 2017)

Websites

Nutritional Information: nutritiondata.self.com

An outstanding, user-friendly website providing detailed nutrition information, plus unique analysis tools that tell you more about how foods affect your health making it easier for you to choose healthy food.

Food Options

Thrive Market: thrivemarket.com

Thrive Market provides you the opportunity to order healthy organic foods and delivers them right to your door.

Vital Choice: vitalchoice.com

Vital Choice sells only sustainably caught seafood. They also support planet-protecting programs and environmental strategies for a healthy Earth by donating a portion of their profits.

Gut Health

SIBO and IBS: thesibodoctor.com

Founder Nirala Jacobi, ND, an expert in SIBO and IBS, provides a lot of resources and recipes, along with a podcast, and provides both patient courses and practitioner training programs as part of her mission to *Beat SIBO and IBS for good.*

Hormone Health

Hormone Balance: hormonesbalance.com

Magdalena Wszelaki is a certified health coach and chef who has a passion for using food as medicine. She has authored two books on how to use food to restore hormone balance. She also has an entire line of natural skincare products called *Wellena*.

Genetics and Your Health

Genetics: strategene.me

Founder Ben Lynch, ND, and author of *Dirty Genes*, provides a one-stop-shop for your genetic testing. DNA saliva sample collection kits are available through seekinghealth.com. Your results package includes educational videos and resources to help you gain a better understanding of the pathways affected by your genes. I encourage you to work with a trained professional when evaluating your genetics and implementing changes.

Environmental Awareness

Environmental Resources: ewg.org

The Environmental Working Group is a valuable resource offering you practical information regarding food safety, personal care, and cosmetics safety, along with home cleaning supplies you can use to protect yourself, your family, and your community

Naturopathic and Integrative Organizations

AANP: naturopathic.org

American Association of Naturopathic Physicians (AANP) is an organization devoted to enhancing human health and wellness by advancing the profession of naturopathic medicine. They provide a listing of Licensed NDs, listed nationally or through their local state organizations.

ACAM: acam.org

American College for Advancement in Medicine (ACAM) is an organization dedicated to bridging the gap between conventional medicine and complementary or alternative medicine.

A4M and IFM: a4m.com and ifm.org

The American Academy of Antiaging and Functional Medicine (A4M) and the Institute for Functional Medicine (IFM) are integrative medicine organizations promoting health and wellness through training and certifying providers on how to empower patients to address the how and why of disease.

AAEM: aaemonline.org

American Academy of Environmental Medicine promotes health by supporting physicians and other professionals in serving the public through education about the interaction between humans and their environment.

NAEM: envmedicine.com

National Association of Environmental Medicine (NAEM) serves as a resource and community for clinicians to learn and lead in the burgeoning field of environmental medicine.

About the Author

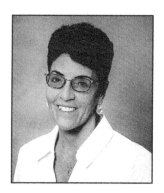

Dr. June Stevens

June E. Stevens, ND, is a clinician, educator, and author who grew up on a family farm in Maine. She has always loved plants and appreciated nature. She served as a registered nurse in the U.S. Navy before pursing her true passion: naturopathic medicine. She received her doctorate from Southwest College of Naturopathic Medicine in Tempe, Arizona; her masters in metabolic and nutritional medicine from the University of South Florida, College of Medicine; and her bachelor's in nursing from the University of Southern Maine.

Dr. Stevens served as an adjunct facility member at the Southwest College of Naturopathic Medicine and was a guest lecturer at the University of Arizona's Center for Integrative Medicine.

As an author, Dr. Stevens was a contributing author for *Prescription for Nutritional Healing*, 4th Ed. Her current book, *What in the Gut Is Going On?*, is the first book in her Naturopathic Wisdom series. As a clinician, Dr. Stevens is owner of NOR CAL Natural Medicine in Redding, California, working primarily in women's health and cardiology.

A subject matter expert in naturopathic and functional approaches to health, Dr. Stevens determines the root cause of her patients' condition, respects their unique biochemical individuality when developing personalized treatment plans, and educates and empowers her patients to become active participants in their healthcare.

Her mission: put *health* back into *healthcare* and move the world toward wellness.

Dr. Stevens lives in Northern California with her spouse, Melanie, and their three dogs: Hillary, Sophie, and Pippa.

For more information visit drjunestevens.com.

Endnotes

Introduction

1 Perlmutter, D. "The GRAIN BRAIN whole life plan." November 14, 2016. https://www.youtube.com/watch?v=BFdaea8fIaU

Chapter One: A Silent Epidemic—Estrogen Dominance

2 Haaland, M. "Nearly half of women have been affected by a hormonal imbalance." *New York Post*. February 22, 2019. https://nypost.com/2019/02/22/nearly-half-of-women-have-been-affected-by-a-hormonal-imbalance/

3 "11 unexpected signs of hormonal imbalance." *Northwell Health*. November 27, 2018. https://www.northwell.edu/obstetrics-and-gynecology/fertility/expert-insights/11-unexpected-signs-of-hormonal-imbalance

4 "Is breast cancer on the rise in young women?" *University of Utah*. August 8, 2019. https://healthcare.utah.edu/the-scope/shows.php?shows=0_61wyemc1

5 Dotinga, R. "PCOS incidence is on the rise, but it remains underdiagnosed and undermanaged." *MDedge*. August 8, 2019. https://www.mdedge.com/clinicianreviews/article/206123/endocrinology/pcos-incidence-rise-it-remains-underdiagnosed-and

6 Ritchie, H., and Roser, M. "Obesity." *Our World in Data*. 2017. https://ourworldindata.org/obesity

7 "Noncommunicable diseases now biggest killers." *World Health Organization*. May 19, 2008. https://www.who.int/mediacentre/news/releases/2008/pr14/en/

8 "About Chronic Diseases." *Centers for Disease Control and Prevention.* 2021. https://www.cdc.gov/chronicdisease/about/index.htm

9 "Five emerging medical specialties you've never heard of—until now." *Association of American Medical Colleges.* 2021. https://www.aamc.org/news-insights/five-emerging-medical-specialties-you-ve-never-heard-until-now

10 Labhart, A. *Clinical Endocrinology: Theory and Practice.* Springer Berlin Heidelberg. December 6, 2012.

11 Lee, J. R. and Hopkins, V. *What Your Doctor May Not Tell You About Menopause: The Breakthrough Book on Natural Progesterone.* Warner Brooks. 1996.

12 "Free and bound T4." *University of Rochester Medical Center.* 2021. https://www.urmc.rochester.edu/encyclopedia/content.aspx?contenttypeid=167&contentid=t4_free_and_bound_blood

13 Laukkarinen, J., *et al.* "The underlying mechanisms: How hypothyroidism affects the formation of common bile duct stones." *HPB Surgery.* September 12, 2012. https://www.ncbi.nlm.nih.gov/pmc/articles/PMC3459253/

14 Want, H. H., *et al.* "New insights into the molecular mechanisms underlying effects of estrogen on cholesterol gallstone formation." *National Institutes of Health.* November 1, 2010. https://www.ncbi.nlm.nih.gov/pmc/articles/PMC2756670/

15 "Estrogen dominance in women." *Naturopathic Doctor News and Review.* February 6, 2019. https://ndnr.com/endocrinology/estrogen-dominance-in-women/

16 Zhu, Y., *et al*. "The toxic effects of xenobiotics on the health of humans and animals." *Hindawi*. March 29, 2017. https://www. hindawi.com/journals/bmri/2017/4627872/

17 Travison, T. G., *et al*. "A population-level decline in serum testosterone levels in American men." *J Clin Endocinal Metab*. January, 2007. https://pubmed.ncbi.nlm.nih.gov/17062768/

18 "Estrogen dominance in men." *Naturopathic Doctor News and Review*. November 5, 2018. https://ndnr.com/mens-health/ estrogen-dominance-in-men/

19 Bosland, M. C. "The role of estrogens in Prostate Carcinogenesis: A rationale for chemoprevention." *Reviews in Urology*. 2005. https://www.ncbi.nlm.nih.gov/pmc/articles/PMC1477605/pdf/ RIU007003_00S4.pdf

20 "The science of saliva testing." *ZRT Laboratory*. February 25, 2014. https://www.zrtlab.com/images/documents/about_saliva_ testing_pds.pdf

21 Kaiser, Wynter. "What does DUTCH test? 4 groups of hormones, metabolites & other biomarkers." *Precision Analytical Inc*. March 2, 2021. https://dutchtest.com/2021/03/02/what-does-dutch-test/

Chapter 2: Your Lymphatics— The Forgotten Detoxification Organ

22 Mitchell, H. H., *et al*. "The chemical composition of the adult human body and its bearing on the biochemistry of growth." *University of Illinois, Urbana*. February 1945. https://bionumbers. hms.harvard.edu/files/625.full.pdf

23 Vighi, G., *et al.* "Allergy and the gastrointestinal system." *Clinical and Experimental Immunology.* September 2008. https://www.ncbi. nlm.nih.gov/pmc/articles/PMC2515351/

Chapter 3: Your Gallbladder and Bile—The Dynamic Duo

24 Latenstein, C., et al. "Etiologies of long-term postcholecystectomy symptoms: A systematic review." *Gastroenterology Research and Practice.* April 2019. https://www. hindawi.com/journals/grp/2019/4278373/

25 Kasbo, J., et al. "Phosphatidylcholine-enriched diet prevents gallstone formation in mice susceptible to cholelithiasis." *Journal of Lipid Research.* December 1, 2003. https://www.jlr.org/article/ S0022-2275(20)31947-7/fulltext

26 Fallingborg, J. "Intraluminal pH of the human gastrointestinal tract." *Dan Med Bull.* June 1999. https://pubmed.ncbi.nlm.nih. gov/?term=%22Dan+Med+Bull%22%5Bjour%5D

27 Chiang, J. Y. "Bile acid metabolism and signaling." *Comprehensive Physiology.* May 2013. https://www.ncbi.nlm.nih.gov/pmc/articles/ PMC4422175/

28 Yasar, C., *et al.* "Impaired gallbladder motility and increased gallbladder wall thickness in patients with nonalcoholic fatty liver disease." *Journal of Neurogastroenterology and Motility.* July 30, 2016. https://www.jnmjournal.org/journal/view.html?doi=10.5056/ jnm15159

29 Yang, Y. C., *et al.* "Long-term Proton Pump Inhibitor Administration Caused Physiological and Microbiota Changes in Rats." *Sci Rep*10, 866. 2020. doi.org/10.1038/s41598-020-57612-8

30 Hoon, L., *et al.* "Parasitic diseases of biliary tract." *American Journal of Roentgenology.* 2007. www.ajronline.org/doi/10.2214/ AJR.06.1172

Chapter 4: Your Liver—The Body's Major Detoxification Organ

31 Environmental Health Symposium 2017. San Diego, California. March 2–5, 2017.

32 Malekinejad, H., and Aysa, R. "Hormones in dairy foods and their impact on public health." *Iranian Journal of Public Health.* February 11, 2015. https://www.ncbi.nlm.nih.gov/pmc/articles/ PMC4524299/

33 Ganmaa D., and Sato, A. "The possible role of female sex hormones in milk from pregnant cows in the development of breast, ovarian and corpus uteri cancers." *Med Hypotheses.* August 24, 2005. https://pubmed.ncbi.nlm.nih.gov/16125328/

34 "Recombinant bovine growth hormone." *American Cancer Society.* September 2014. https://www.cancer.org/cancer/cancer-causes/ recombinant-bovine-growth-hormone.html

35 "Questions and answers: summary report on antimicrobials sold or distributed for use in food-producing animals." *U.S. Food and Drug Administration.* 2020. https://www.fda.gov/industry/ animal-drug-user-fee-act-adufa/questions-and-answers-summary-report-antimicrobials-sold-or-distributed-use-food-producing-animals

36 "FDA releases annual summary report on antimicrobials sold or distributed in 2018 for use in food-producing animals." *U.S. Food and Drug Administration.* December 10, 2019. https://www.fda. gov/animal-veterinary/cvm-updates/fda-releases-annual-summary-report-antimicrobials-sold-or-distributed-2018-use-food-producing

37 Fucic, A., *et al.* "Environmental exposure to xenoestrogens and oestrogen related cancers: reproductive system, breast, lung, kidney, pancreas, and brain." *Environmental health: a global access science source.* 2012. https://www.ncbi.nlm.nih.gov/pmc/articles/PMC3388472/

38 Teng, Y., *et al.* "Plant-derived exosomal microRNAs shape the gut microbiota." *Cell Host Microbe.* October 25, 2018. https://pubmed.ncbi.nlm.nih.gov/30449315/

39 Helferich, W. G., *et al.* "Phytoestrogens and breast cancer: a complex story." *Inflammopharmacology.* October 16, 2008. https://pubmed.ncbi.nlm.nih.gov/18815740/

40 "What are high-risk crops and inputs?" *Non-GMO Project.* 2020. https://www.nongmoproject.org/gmo-facts/high-risk/

41 Robinson, C., and Perro, M. "Glyphosate and Roundup disrupt the gut microbiome by inhibiting the shikimate pathway." *GMOScience.* February 20, 2020. https://www.gmoscience.org/glyphosate-and-roundup-disrupt-the-gut-microbiome-by-inhibiting-the-shikimate-pathway/

42 Hodges, R. E., and Minich, D. M. "Modulation of metabolic detoxification pathways using foods and food-derived components: A scientific review with clinical application." *Journal of Nutrition and Metabolism.* 2015. https://doi.org/10.1155/2015/760689

43 Magnesium: Fact sheet for health professionals." *National Institutes of Health.* https://ods.od.nih.gov/factsheets/Magnesium-HealthProfessional/#en10

44 "2015–2020 dietary guidelines for Americans." *U.S. Department of Health and Human Services and US Department of Agriculture.* December 2015. https://health.gov/dietaryguidelines/2015/

45 Wallace T. C., *et al.* "Multivitamin/mineral supplement contribution to micronutrient intakes in the United States 2007-2010." *J Am Coll Nutr.* 2014. https://www.ncbi.nlm.nih.gov/pubmed/24724766

46 Alegría-Torres, J. A., *et al.* "Epigenetics and lifestyle." *Epigenomics.* 2011. https://doi.org/10.2217/epi.11.22

47 Tsao, D., *et al.* "Serotonin-induced hypersensitivity via inhibition of catechol O-methyltransferase activity." *Molecular Pain.* January 1, 2012. https://doi.org/10.1186/1744-8069-8-25

48 Lynch, D. *Dirty Genes.* HarperOne. 2018. 77.

49 Halderman, K. "Phase 2.5 detox with Dr. Kelly Halderman." *Viva Natural Health*, YouTube. November 8, 2020. https://www.youtube.com/watch?v=yBrUUZiaNVA

50 Pizzino, G., *et al.* "Oxidative stress: Harms and benefits for human health." *Oxidative medicine and cellular longevity.* 2017. https://doi.org/10.1155/2017/8416763

51 Wessler, J. D., *et al.* "The P-glycoprotein transport system and cardiovascular drugs." *ScienceDirect.* June 2013. https://www.sciencedirect.com/science/article/pii/S0735109713012916#tbl1fndagger

52 Kapoor, A., *et al.* "Effects of sertraline and fluoxetine on p-glycoprotein at barrier sites: In vivo and in vitro approaches." *PloS One.* 2013. https://www.ncbi.nlm.nih.gov/pmc/articles/PMC3585317/

53 Ruike, Z., *et al.* "In vitro and in vivo evaluation of the effects of duloxetine on P-gp function." *Human Psychopharmacology.* February 11, 2011. https://doi.org/10.1002/hup.1152

54 Xie, Y., *et al.* "Risk of death among users of proton pump inhibitors: A longitudinal observational cohort study of United States veterans." *BMJ Open.* 2017. https://bmjopen.bmj.com/content/7/6/e015735.citation-tools

Chapter 5: Your Gut Microbiome

55 Sender, R., *et al.* "Revised estimates for the number of human and bacteria cells in the body. *PLoS Biology.* 2016. https://doi.org/10.1371/journal.pbio.1002533

56 McBurney, M. I. "Establishing what constitutes a healthy human gut microbiome: State of the science, regulatory considerations, and future directions." *The Journal of Nutrition.* November 2019. https://doi.org/10.1093/jn/nxz154

57 Eisenstein, M. "The hunt for a healthy microbiome." *Nature.* January 29, 2020. https://www.nature.com/articles/d41586-020-00193-3#:~:text=Some%20500%E2%80%931%2C000%20bacterial%20species,viruses%2C%20fungi%20and%20other%20microbes

58 Thursby, E., and Juge, N. "Introduction to the human gut microbiota." *The Biochemical Journal.* 2017. https://doi.org/10.1042/BCJ20160510

59 Hodges, R. E., and Minich, D. M. "Modulation of metabolic detoxification pathways using foods and food-derived components: A scientific review with clinical application. *Journal of Nutrition and Metabolism.* 2015. https://doi.org/10.1155/2015/760689

60 Patterson, R., and Sears, D. "Metabolic effects of intermittent fasting." *Annual Reviews.* 2017. https://www.annualreviews.org/doi/full/10.1146/annurev-nutr-071816-

064634?url_ver=Z39.88-2003&rfr_id=ori%3Arid%3Acrossref.
org&rfr_dat=cr_pub%3Dpubmed

Chapter 6: The Removal and Replacement Process

61 "Noncommunicable diseases." *World Health Organization*. April
13, 2021. https://www.who.int/news-room/fact-sheets/detail/
noncommunicable-diseases

62 "The inside story: a guide to indoor air quality." *United States
Environmental Protection Agency*. 2020. https://www.epa.gov/indoor-
air-quality-iaq/inside-story-guide-indoor-air-quality#main-content

63 Sholl, J. "8 hidden toxins: What's lurking in your cleaning
products?" *Experience Life*. October 2011. https://experiencelife.
lifetime.life/article/8-hidden-toxins-whats-lurking-in-your-
cleaning-products/

64 Sharma, A. *et al*. "E-cigarettes compromise the gut barrier
and trigger inflammation." iScience. Jan 6, 2021. https://doi.
org/10.1016/j.isci.2021.102035

65 Hauck, Z. "The effects cannabis on your hormones." *The ZRT
Laboratory Blog*. June 20, 2019. https://www.zrtlab.com/blog/
archive/the-effects-of-cannabis-on-your-hormones/#B1

66 Carr, T. "Too many meds? America's love affair with prescription
medication." *Consumer Reports*. August 3, 2017. https://www.
consumerreports.org/prescription-drugs/too-many-meds-americas-
love-affair-with-prescription-medication/#nation

67 Ramirex, J. *et al*. "Antibiotics as Major Disruptors of Gut
Microbiota." *Frontiers in Cellular and Infection Microbiology*. 24
November 2020. https://doi.org/10.3389/fcimb.2020.572912

68 Bethesda (MD). "Estrogens and oral contraceptive." *LiverTox: Clinical and Research Information on Drug-Induced Liver Injury*. National Institute of Diabetes and Digestive and Kidney Diseases. 2012. https://www.ncbi.nlm.nih.gov/books/NBK548539/

69 Buschman, H. "Big data from world's largest citizen science microbiome project serves food for thought." *UC San Diego Health*. May 15, 2018. https://health.ucsd.edu/news/releases/Pages/2018-05-15-big-data-from-worlds-largest-citizen-science-microbiome-project-serves-food-for-thought.aspx

70 Cabbage Town Pet Clinic. "How Essential Oils Can Affect Your Pet's Health." March 2, 2020. cabbagetownpetclinic.com/2020/03/02/how-essential-oils-can-affect-your-pets-health/

71 "Personal care products safety act would improve cosmetics safety." Environmental Working Group. 2020. https://www.ewg.org/personal-care-products-safety-act-would-improve-cosmetics-safety

72 "Dietary Guidelines for Alcohol." *Centers for Disease Control and Prevention*. December 29, 2020. https://www.cdc.gov/alcohol/fact-sheets/moderate-drinking.htm

73 Hauck, Z. "The effects cannabis on your hormones." *The ZRT Laboratory Blog*. June 20, 2019. https://www.zrtlab.com/blog/archive/the-effects-of-cannabis-on-your-hormones/#B1

74 Omecare. "The Genetics Behind Your Caffeine Consumption." July 2020. omecare.com/resources/blog/the-genetics-behind-your-caffeine-consumption/

75 "Spilling the beans: How much caffeine is too much?" *U.S. Food & Drug Administration*. December 12, 2018. https://www.fda.gov/consumers/consumer-updates/spilling-beans-how-much-caffeine-too-much

Chapter 7: Liberate Your Lymphatics

76 Bhattacharya, A., *et al.* "Body acceleration distribution and O2 uptake in humans during running and jumping." *Journal of Applied Psychology*. 1980. https://pubmed.ncbi.nlm.nih.gov/7429911/

77 "America's #1 Health Problem." *The American Institute of Stress*. 2020. https://www.stress.org/americas-1-health-problem

Chapter 8: Build Your Bile

78 "Increasing fiber intake." *University of California San Francisco*. 2020. https://www.ucsfhealth.org/education/increasing-fiber-intake

79 Zeisel, S. H., and Costas, K. A. "Choline: an essential nutrient for public health." *Nutrition reviews*. 2009. https://doi.org/10.1111/j.1753-4887.2009.00246.x

80 Dagfinn, A., *et al.* "Physical activity and the risk of gallbladder disease: A systematic review and meta-analysis of cohort studies." *Journal of Physical Activity, and Health*. 2016. https://doi.org/10.1123/jpah.2015-0456

81 Reynolds, A. N., *et al.* "Advice to walk after meals is more effective for lowering postprandial glycaemia in type 2 diabetes mellitus than advice that does not specify timing: a randomised crossover study." *Diabetologia*. October 17, 2016. https://link.springer.com/article/10.1007/s00125-016-4085-2

82 Early, R. L., *et al.* "The gall of subordination: changed in gallbladder function associated with social stress." *The Royal Society*. November 24, 2003. https://www.ncbi.nlm.nih.gov/pmc/articles/PMC1691567/pdf/15002765.pdf

83 "2015–2016 dietary guidelines." *Health.gov*. 2015. https://health.gov/our-work/food-nutrition/previous-dietary-guidelines/2015

84 "Choline: fact sheet for health professionals." *National Institutes of Health.* 2020. https://ods.od.nih.gov/factsheets/Choline-HealthProfessional/#h2

Chapter 9: Love Your Liver

85 Panieri, E., *et al.* "Potential applications of NRF2 modulators in cancer therapy." *Antioxidants (Basel, Switzerland).* 2020. https://doi.org/10.3390/antiox9030193

86 Johnson, C. "Putting the puzzle pieces of phase 1, 2, and 3 estrogen detoxification together." *Precision Analytical.* November 5, 2018. https://www.youtube.com/watch?v=Zsga25I9PG4&t=3143s

Chapter 10: Maximize Your Microbiome

87 Feltman, R. "The gut's microbiome changes rapidly with diet: A new study finds that populations of bacteria in the gut are highly sensitive to the food we digest." *Scientific American.* December 14, 2013. https://www.scientificamerican.com/article/the-guts-microbiome-changes-diet/#

88 Li, Y., *et al.* "The role of microbiome in insomnia, circadian disturbance and depression." *Frontiers in psychiatry.* 2018. https://doi.org/10.3389/fpsyt.2018.00669

89 Bressa, C., *et al.* "Differences in gut microbiota profile between women with active lifestyle and sedentary women." *PloS one.* 2017. https://doi.org/10.1371/journal.pone.0171352

90 Caminero, A., *et al.* "Mechanisms by which gut microorganisms influence food sensitivities." *Nature Reviews Gastroenterology and Hepatology.* 2019. https://doi.org/10.1038/s41575-018-0064-z

91 Born, T. A. "Topical Use of Castor Oil." *Naturopathic News and Review*. May 5, 2015. https://ndnr.com/dermatology/topical-use-of-castor-oil/

92 Grady, H. "Immunomodulation through castor oil packs." *Journal of Naturopathic Medicine*. 1999. https://drprincetta.com/wp-content/uploads/2016/01/Castor-Oil-Packs-Immunomodulation.pdf

93 Gerson, M. "The cure of advanced cancer by diet therapy: a summary of 30 years of clinical experimentation." *Physiological chemistry and physics*. 1974. https://pubmed.ncbi.nlm.nih.gov/751079/

94 Teekachunhatean, S. *et al.* "Pharmacokinetics of Caffeine Following a Single . . ." *ISRN Pharmacol*. Mar 4, 2013. DOI: 10.1155/2013/147238

Appendix B: Supplementation Support

95 "A. G. Schneiderman asks major retailers to halt sales of certain herbal supplements as DNA tests fail to detect plant materials listed on majority of products tested." *The New York State Office of the Attorney General*. February 13, 2015. https://ag.ny.gov/press-release/2015/ag-schneiderman-asks-major-retailers-halt-sales-certain-herbal-supplements-dna

96 "FDA takes action against 17 companies for illegally selling products claiming to treat Alzheimer's disease." *U.S. Food and Drug Administration*. February 11, 2019. https://www.fda.gov/news-events/press-announcements/fda-takes-action-against-17-companies-illegally-selling-products-claiming-treat-alzheimers-disease

97 Tigner, S. *Herbal Medicine: From the Heart of the Earth*. Wise Acres Publishing. 1999.

Made in the USA
Las Vegas, NV
06 January 2025

15962683R00154